Essentials
of the
Roy Adaptation
Model

Essentials of the Roy Adaptation Model

Heather A. Andrews
Athabasca University

Sister Callista Roy
University of California

 APPLETON-CENTURY-CROFTS/NORWALK, CONNECTICUT

1986

0-8385-2271-8

88 89 90 / 10 9 8 7 6 5

Prentice-Hall International (UK) Limited, *London*
Prentice-Hall of Australia Pty. Limited, *Sydney*
Editora Prentice-Hall do Brasil, Ltda., *Rio de Janeiro*
Prentice-Hall Canada Inc., *Toronto*
Prentice-Hall Hispanoamericana, S.A., *Mexico*
Prentice-Hall of India Private Limited, *New Delhi*
Prentice-Hall of Japan, Inc., *Tokyo*
Prentice-Hall of Southeast Asia Pte. Ltd., *Singapore*
Whitehall Books Limited, *Wellington, New Zealand*

Library of Congress Cataloging-in-Publication Data
Andrews, Heather A.
  Essentials of the Roy Adaptation Model.

  Based on the 1984 edition of Introduction to
nursing by Callista Roy.
  Includes bibliographies and index.
  1. Nursing—Psychological aspects. 2. Nurses—
Psychology. 3. Nurse and patient. I. Roy, Callista.
II. Introduction to nurisng. III. Title.
RT86.A52 1986   610.73'019   85-3533
ISBN 0-8385-2271-8 (Appleton-Century-Crofts)

Editorial/production supervision and
  interior design: Maria McColligan
Cover design: Ben Santora
Manufacturing buyer: John B. Hall

PRINTED IN THE UNITED STATES OF AMERICA

Contents

Preface

Essentials of the Roy Adaptation Model is an introduction to the Adaptation Model for nursing developed by Sister Callista Roy. Its purpose is to highlight the essential elements of the model and to provide an overview and brief description of the key concepts.

Although textbooks on nursing models in general and the Adaptation Model specifically have become increasingly available, there is an identified need for a book that presents the major concepts of an established and implemented model for nursing practice at a basic level. This book focuses on the essential elements of one such model. It presents the elements of the Roy Adaptation Model in a clear, concise, and basic manner with emphasis on the nursing process and its application in practice. This text features a dynamic visual depiction of the concepts through a diagrammatic representation of the model.

Based on the 1984 edition of *Introduction to Nursing: An Adaptation Model* by Sister Roy, the discussion emphasizes Roy's description of the key elements of nursing models: the person, environment, health, and nursing. Particular emphasis is placed on the person and nursing activities. A brief introduction to the model's four adaptive modes is also included.

The relationships in the model are illustrated by a diagrammatic conceptualization of the model that was developed at the Royal Alexandra Hospitals School of Nursing, Edmonton, Alberta, Canada, during the time the nursing curriculum was being restructured based on the Roy Model. This visual representation of the model has proven to be an effective teaching tool.

Specific objectives are provided at the beginning of each chapter to enable the reader to focus on key concepts and to assist in the achievement of understanding. Illustrations and examples apply the concepts to common life situations, while exercises for application allow the reader to apply further the concepts to described situations. Questions and feedback at the end of each chapter provide for assessment of understanding and attainment of the previously identified objectives. Introductions and summaries in each chapter provide an overview and review of the content. For readers requiring supplementary material, references are given.

This text is intended primarily for use in agencies or educational institutions that are using the Roy Adaptation Model as a basis for nursing practice and education. It is often necessary to provide individuals, new students in diploma or associate degree programs, for example, with an overview of the model before more in-depth study can begin. The text could also be a useful orientation tool for nursing service personnel and faculty.

For those considering the incorporation of the Roy Adaptation Model into their educational program or practice setting, this description provides an efficient method to become acquainted with the essentials. In addition, the text is a useful resource for those nurses in baccalaureate or master level programs undertaking a general study of nursing models.

It is becoming increasingly necessary to articulate the unique perspective and role of nursing and nurses to other professionals in the interdisciplinary health team. It is hoped that this text will assist in this important, but sometimes difficult, task.

The authors are indebted to many people for their encouragement and assistance in the development of this text. First, we acknowledge those who have contributed to and offered stimulation for the current level of development of the Roy Adaptation Model. Particularly, we are grateful to the faculty and students of Mount St. Mary's College and to the graduate students throughout the world who communicate with Sister Callista. The faculty and students of the Royal Alexandra Hospitals School of Nursing had a special role in developing and testing earlier presentations of the essentials of the model. Particular recognition and appreciation is given to Gloria Bauer, Director of this school of nursing, for her tangible support and encouragement throughout the project and to Myrna Doell who capably handled the typing of the manuscript. The direction and skill provided by our production editor, Maria McColligan, contributed greatly to the presentation of our work. Family, friends, and colleagues have contributed to the project in ways that they may not even recognize.

The authors share responsibility for the content and quality of the text. However, Sister Callista acknowledges the leadership taken by Mrs. Andrews in developing the project and applying her skills as an educator to contribute greatly to the clarity of the presentation. Her ability to develop the working relationship of a close colleague with Sister Callista over barriers of distance and competing demands helped bring this book into publication. We also thank Maureen Jakocko and Linda Sowden for sharing their experience with the Roy Model in practice in Chapter 16.

This book is presented with the hope and belief that it will contribute to the quality with which the practice of nursing is learned and to the scientific and humanistic basis of nursing care.

Heather A. Andrews

Sister Callista Roy

Part I

Introduction to the Roy Adaptation Model

The Roy Adaptation Model is currently one of the most highly developed and widely used conceptual descriptions of nursing. Formal development of the model began in the late 1960s and, since that time, nurses in the United States and around the world have helped Roy in clarifying, refining, and extending the basic concepts to the stage of development presented in this text. In addition to addressing nursing models in general, the following chapter provides a cursory overview of the major concepts addressed in all nursing models—person, environment, health, and nursing—as described in the Roy Adaptation Model. Each of these is discussed in greater depth in subsequent chapters of this text.

Chapter 1

Overview of the Roy Adaptation Model

Nurses use special knowledge to help promote and restore health. This chapter introduces nursing's special knowledge by describing models for nursing practice and by providing an overview of one particular model, the Roy Adaptation Model for Nursing.

Models for nursing have developed rapidly over the past few decades and even the beginning nurse will want to be informed about this advance in the science of nursing. In addition, every practicing nurse will want her nursing care to be based upon a clear understanding of what nursing is and the service that it provides.

OBJECTIVES

After studying this chapter, the reader should be able to do the following:

1. Describe a nursing model.
2. Identify the major parts of a nursing model.
3. Identify the key terms in Roy's description of the person.
4. Recognize Roy's definition of the environment.
5. Define health according to the Roy Adaptation Model.
6. Identify the six steps of nursing as described in the Roy Adaptation Model.

NURSING MODELS

A model is a representation that helps us understand the thing it represents. For example, a model home allows the person considering buying a home to become familiar with layout of the rooms of a particular house that is not yet built. Similarly, in the lobbies of hospitals one frequently sees a scale model showing the building being planned to enlarge the agency. In this way, one sees all the parts of the thing represented and the relationships of those parts to each other. In the example of the hospital building plans, one sees a new emergency room and outpatient department. The expansion of parking facilities is indicated and one can identify how each of these parts relates to the other and to the buildings and other parking lots already standing.

Nurses have been building models to represent the reality of nursing as they see it for over one hundred years. A model of nursing can be defined as a representation of the major parts of nursing and how these relate to one another. When scholars read the works of nurses, they observe that, since the time of Florence Nightingale (1859), the major writers have described four concepts that are the essential parts of nursing. These four parts are (1) **person**, (2) **environment**, (3) **nursing**, and (4) **health**.

Any science has its own view of the reality that it studies. Although physiologists and psychologists both study human brain function, physiology focuses on the vital processes of a living organism while psychology focuses on human behavior aspects. As a science, nursing has been developing a unique way of viewing the person in relation to the environment and how nursing interacts with the person to promote health within this environment. Various authors place different emphasis on each of these parts and define them somewhat differently. Certain commonalities can be seen in writings about the science of nursing and how it describes persons, environment, nursing, and health.

Nursing views *persons* as holistic and developing beings with the processes and capacity for thinking, feeling, reflecting, and choosing. Human behavior has pattern and meaning. Persons respond to and act upon everything that is within and around them. The term *environment* is used to describe the world within and around the person. *Nursing* acts to enhance the interaction of the person within this environment. The goal is to promote growth and meaningful life for the individual in harmony with his or her social and physical environment. In this way, nursing promotes health. *Health*, then, is a function of human and environmental patterns that enhance one another and that express full life potential for the person.

When the nurse is caring for a person, it makes a difference how she[1] views the nature of human beings. If she considers the person holistically, she cannot simply treat his fractured leg. At the same time she sees that the person is frightened by the surgery scheduled to reduce the fracture and is feeling lonely because the accident in which he was injured happened at a distance from home. Believing in the person's ability to reflect upon experience and to choose, the nurse recognizes that she can help him to respond to his experience in a positive way. A nurse's practice is greatly influenced by the way she sees the essential parts of nursing.

Although the person is the key concept of nursing, nursing practice is influenced by the nurse's view of the other parts described in nursing models. For example, if the nurse sees the person and environment as mutually enhancing instead of in opposition, then she can assist persons to interact positively with the world around them. For example, she can make it possible for the lonely person awaiting surgery to visit with other patients. Similarly, the nurse who sees her role in the broad sense of promoting growth and health will be less likely to focus solely on technical skills. And if she recognizes that health involves expression of full life potential, the nurse can promote the health of terminally ill persons by helping them to fully express who they are in this final act of life as we know it.

Nursing models, then, provide a representation of how particular nurses describe nursing science's view of persons, environment, nursing, and health. During the decades of the 1970s and 1980s, nurse authors have written extensively about these major concepts of nursing. Each model, or representation of the major parts of nursing, has been useful in clarifying what nursing is and the service that nurses can provide. Furthermore, nursing models have led to the more systematic development of nursing knowledge as the scientific basis for nursing practice. A number of texts are available that describe each of these models in greater detail. (See, for example, Riehl and Roy 1980; Fitzpatrick and Whall 1983.)

THE ROY ADAPTATION MODEL

The Roy Adaptation Model is one of the most highly developed and widely used models. This text focuses on this specific model for nursing practice. The major concepts of the model—person, environment,

---

[1] It is recognized that nurses are both male and female. Feminine pronouns are used throughout this text to refer to the nurse to simplify presentation.

nursing, and health—are introduced in this chapter and discussed in greater detail throughout the book. In addition, the reader is referred to the definitive works on this model by its original author. (See particularly Roy 1984; Roy and Roberts 1981.)

Historical Development

The first formal descriptions of the Roy Adaptation Model were made by Sister Callista Roy while she was a graduate student in the School of Nursing at the University of California at Los Angeles. The roots of the model lie in Roy's own personal and professional background. Roy is committed to a philosophical belief in the innate capabilities, purpose, and worth of the human person. Her clinical practice in pediatric nursing provided experience with the resiliency of the human body and spirit. Under the mentorship of Dorothy E. Johnson, Roy became convinced of the importance of defining nursing. She was influenced also by her studies in the social sciences. She began to seek ways to express her beliefs about nursing and to explore these further in her studies. Her first publication on the Roy Adaptation Model appeared in 1970. (See Roy 1970.) By that time, Roy was on the faculty of the baccalaureate nursing program of a small liberal arts college. There she had the opportunity to lead the implementation of this model of nursing as the basis of the nursing curriculum. During the next decade, more than 1500 faculty and students at Mount St. Mary's College helped to clarify, refine, and extend the basic concepts of the Roy Adaptation Model for Nursing.

First Major Concept—Person

As noted earlier, the first major concept of a nursing model is person. The nurse describes a particular view of the human person that differs from that of the other sciences. Nurses care for persons as individuals and for persons in groups. For example, one nurse may be preparing a young man for surgery the next day and another nurse may be providing emergency aid to victims and dealing with survivors, witnesses, and family members at the site of a disaster. According to the Roy Adaptation Model, the person as an individual and as a member of a group is described as an **adaptive system.**

As with any system, the person takes in input and processes this input to produce a response, or output. Roy's early notion was that human behavior could be viewed as the output of the adaptive system. The behavior might be adaptive for the person or ineffective. **Adaptive behavior** is evidence of effective response to stimuli while **ineffective**

behavior indicates problems. In studying adaptation further, Roy described the factors that affect whether the behavior is adaptive or ineffective. The person's behavior is influenced both by the environment, that is, the world within and around the person, and by the person's abilities to deal with that world. A simple example of the person responding as an adaptive system is the decision to return to school to prepare for a new career. This decision may be a response to the external circumstances of a changing economy and technology that makes the person's current skills outdated. In addition, it is influenced by the person's usual motivation and ability to problem solve and to find new ways to deal with the task of making a living.

Roy has described the environmental input for the person as stimuli that may be focal, contextual, or residual. The person's **coping mechanisms** for dealing with the world are broadly categorized as the **regulator subsystem** or the **cognator subsystem**. Regulator coping mechanisms respond automatically through neural, chemical, and endocrine activity while cognator coping mechanisms respond through cognitive-emotive channels. The behaviors that result from the regulator and cognator mechanisms can be observed in four categories. Roy noted that a large sample of patient behaviors could be categorized according to whether they took place in the **physiological mode, self-concept mode, role function mode**, or **interdependence mode**. She called these categories **adaptive modes** and described them as ways of coping that show the activity of the regulator and cognator mechanisms.

In summary, Roy describes the person as an adaptive system with regulator and cognator mechanisms that act through the four adaptive modes to produce adaptive responses to the changing world within and around. The concept of the person as an adaptive system is explored in more detail in Chapter 2.

Second Major Concept—Environment

Environment is the second major concept of a nursing model and is understood as the world within and around the person. According to the Roy Adaptation Model for Nursing, the changing environment stimulates the person to make adaptive responses. For human beings, life is never the same. It is constantly changing and presenting new challenges. The person has the ability to make new responses to these changing conditions. As the environment changes, the person has the opportunity to continue to grow and develop and to enhance the meaning of life for self and others. One example of a positive response to changing circumstances is the patient who reorders his priorities in life after suffering a near-fatal heart attack. He finds that altering his style of living can provide a more satisfying life for himself and his family.

He decides to spend more of his time and energy with his wife and children and less at work.

In describing the environment, Roy has drawn upon the work of Helson (1964). This physiological psychologist defines *adaptation* as a function of the degree of change taking place and the person's adaptation level. Three types of stimuli pool to make up the person's adaptation level. Those immediately confronting the person are termed **focal stimuli**. All other stimuli present that can be identified as influencing the current situation are called **contextual stimuli**. The **residual stimuli** are those that may influence the adaptation level, but whose effect has not been confirmed.

According to Roy, then, environment includes all conditions, circumstances, and influences surrounding and affecting the development and behavior of the person. These influencing factors are categorized as focal, contextual, and residual stimuli. Further discussion of these three types of stimuli and how they affect adaptation level can be found in Chapter 3.

Third Major Concept—Health

The third major concept of the model, health, is derived from an understanding of the first two concepts, person and environment. The person is recognized as an adaptive system constantly growing and developing within a changing environment. Roy believes that each person has a unique purpose in life and the potential for fulfilling that purpose. Becoming an integrated and whole person reflects the fulfillment of one's purpose in life. Thus, Roy defines *health* as a state and a process of being and becoming an integrated and whole person. A whole person is one with the highest possible fulfillment of human potential. One can easily recognize a lack of integration as a lack of health. In the example cited earlier, the man who had an imbalance in his work and family life was unhealthy even before he suffered the heart attack.

In the development of the Roy Adaptation Model, the concept of health has been the last of the four concepts to be explored by Roy. This beginning work and its relationship to adaptation as a goal of nursing will be included in Chapter 5.

Fourth Major Concept—Nursing

Based on the other three parts of the model, Roy has developed the fourth concept, nursing. *Nursing* has been described earlier as a science and the application of knowledge from that science to the practice of nursing. The Roy Adaptation Model for Nursing provides a basis for the development of nursing science and a guideline for nursing practice. Discussions of the science of nursing based on this model can be found elsewhere. (See Roy 1984; Roy and Roberts 1981.) The specific activities that distinguish nursing from other disciplines are collectively termed **the nursing process.** This process, according to the Roy Adaptation Model for Nursing, has six steps to problem solving. As a guide to nursing practice, the Roy Model gives specific direction to each step of the nursing process.

Nursing **assessment** means gathering data about the person receiving nursing care. The Roy Adaptation Model has a two-level assessment. In **assessment of behavior,** the nurse identifies patient behavior, that is, how the person is behaving as an adaptive system. Then she moves on to **assessment of stimuli** and notes the factors or stimuli that are affecting that behavior. Based on the assessment information in the first two steps, the nurse makes a statement about the person's adaptive state; this third step of the nursing process is called the **nursing diagnosis.** When an accurate assessment and diagnosis have been made, the nurse plans her care by **goal setting** related to promoting patient adaptation, step four. In the fifth step, she selects and carries out nursing **interventions** that manage the patient's stimuli to promote adaptation. **Evaluation** is the sixth and final step of the nursing process. In this step the nurse determines whether or not the planned interventions have been successful in reaching the goal that she has set with the patient. Each step of the nursing process is described in detail in the six chapters of Part III.

SUMMARY

In this chapter we have looked at nursing models and how they provide representations of the reality of nursing by describing the major components of nursing—person, environment, nursing, and health. A brief overview of the Roy Adaptation Model for Nursing was given so that the reader may be prepared to study this model in greater depth in the chapters that follow.

To illustrate the use of the Roy Adaptation Model, let us describe a common life experience. A young woman is in the process of moving into her first apartment where she plans to live while she is finishing her senior year in college. The behaviors that the neighbors note are that she has brought simple furniture that is in good repair, that several friends help her move into the building, and that she looks tired and hot while she is working. After talking with her for a few minutes, the person in the next apartment recognizes that the young woman has been working hard for several days to get ready for the move, that she and her friends have been driving for several hours to arrive at the new place, and that she had finished her summer job just that week. Furthermore, it is very hot and humid and the air conditioner and elevator at the apartment building are not working. Based on this assessment of the young woman's state of adaptation and the factors influencing it, the neighbor plans to serve lemonade on the patio to her and her friends before they complete the task of moving the furniture.

EXERCISES FOR APPLICATION

1. Suggest several models with which you are familiar that provide a representation of an actual entity. For example, the layout of a model railway may actually represent a segment of a specific rail line. Model airplanes with the same external features of their life-size counterparts may actually be capable of flight.
2. Consider your own beliefs about the four parts of a nursing model: person, environment, nursing, and health. How do they compare with those of Roy as described in this chapter?

ASSESSMENT OF UNDERSTANDING

Questions
1. Which of the following statements apply (applies) to *nursing models*?
   (a) They represent the major parts of nursing.
   (b) They describe how the parts of nursing relate to each other.
   (c) They guide systematic development of nursing knowledge.
2. There are four major concepts or parts included in a description of any nursing model. List them in the spaces provided below.
   (a) _____
   (b) _____
   (c) _____
   (d) _____
3. The following descriptions apply to Roy's view of the person as a major nursing concept. Match the terms on the left with the appropriate description on the right.
   1. Person
   2. Stimuli
   3. Coping mechanisms
   4. Behavior
   5. Adaptive modes

   (a) _____ Focal, contextual, residual
   (b) _____ Adaptive or ineffective responses
   (c) _____ An adaptive system
   (d) _____ Four categories of behavior
   (e) _____ Demonstrate regulator and cognator activity

(f) _____ Environmental input

(g) _____ Regulator and cognator

4. The following definition represents Roy's view of one of the four major concepts commonly addressed in nursing models. Which concept is being addressed?

_____ includes all conditions, circumstances, and influences surrounding and affecting the development and behavior of the person.

5. Fill in the missing words in the following statement pertaining to the third major concept, health.

According to Roy, health is defined as a _____ and _____ of being and becoming an _____ and _____ person.

6. Roy has described the nursing process as six steps to problem solving. The following figure illustrates how these activities can be visually depicted in a circle. In the spaces provided in the circle, insert the appropriate label for each step indicated.

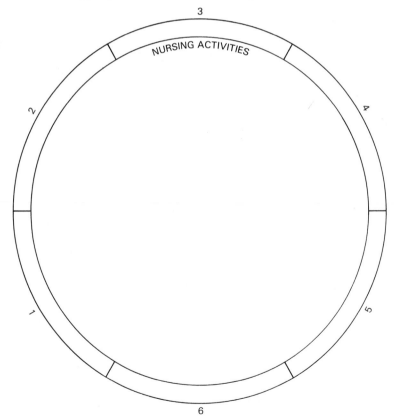

Feedback
1. a, b, c
2. (a) Persons
   (b) Environment
   (c) Nursing
   (d) Health
3. (a) 2
   (b) 4
   (c) 1
   (d) 5
   (e) 5
   (f) 2
   (g) 3
4. Environment
5. State, process, integrated, whole
6.

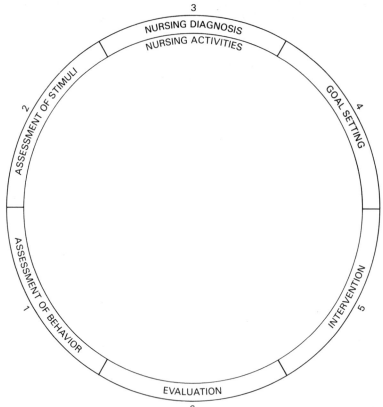

REFERENCES

Fitzpatrick, Joyce J., and Ann L. Whall. *Conceptual Models of Nursing: Analysis and Application.* Bowie, Maryland: Brody Co., 1983.

Helson, Harry. *Adaptation Level Theory.* New York: Harper & Row, Publishers, 1964.

Nightingale, Florence. *Notes of Nursing: What It Is and What It Is Not.* Facsimile of the first edition printed in London, 1859, with a foreword by Annie W. Goodrich. Philadelphia: J. B. Lippincott Co., 1966.

Riehl, Joan P., and Sister Callista Roy. *Conceptual Models for Nursing Practice* (2nd ed.). New York: Appleton-Century-Crofts, 1980.

Roy, Sister Callista. "Adaptation: A Conceptual Framework for Nursing," *Nursing Outlook*, 18, no. 3 (March 1970): 43–45.

———. *Introduction to Nursing: An Adaptation Model* (2nd ed.). Englewood Cliffs, N.J.: Prentice-Hall, Inc., 1984.

Roy, Sister Callista, and Sharon Roberts. *Theory Construction in Nursing: An Adaptation Model.* Englewood Cliffs, N.J.: Prentice-Hall, Inc., 1981.

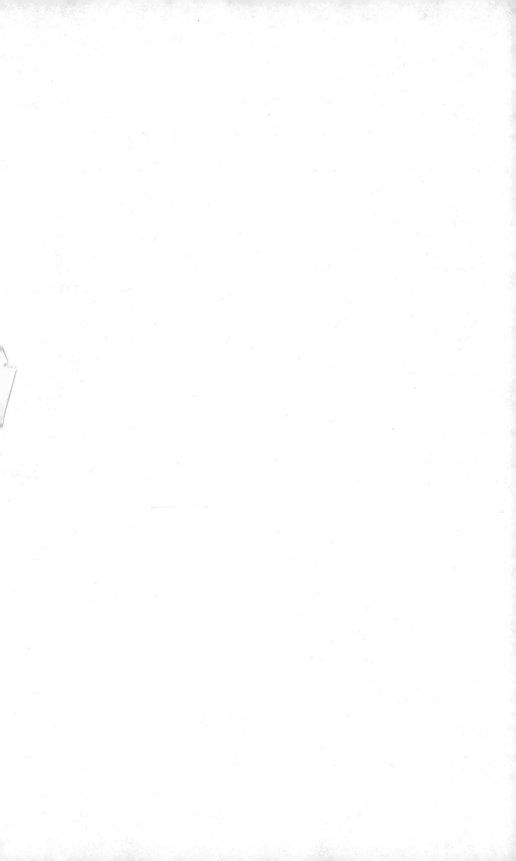

Part II

Major Concepts of the Roy Adaptation Model

In the Roy Adaptation Model for Nursing, the recipient of nursing care is viewed as a holistic adaptive system. The discussion in the following four chapters will focus on Roy's way of viewing the essence of nursing and will highlight the following major concepts: the person as an adaptive system; stimuli, adaptation level, and responses; coping mechanisms and adaptive modes; and the goal of nursing and health. These concepts provide the background for and the basis for the nursing process as viewed by the Roy Adaptation Model.

Chapter 2

The Person as an Adaptive System

The elements of the Roy Adaptation Model for Nursing were discussed briefly in the first chapter. This chapter deals with Roy's view of the person as the recipient of nursing care and the meaning of the words **holistic adaptive system** which are used to describe the individual.

Nursing focuses on persons whether they are sick or well; whether they present individually or as a group. It is necessary for the nurse to have a clear perception and understanding of whom she is dealing with in order to achieve consistency and effectiveness in the nursing care provided.

OBJECTIVES

After studying this chapter, the reader should be able to do the following:

1. Describe Roy's view of the recipient of nursing care.
2. Define *system.*
3. Given an example of a simple system, explain the relationships of input, control, output, and feedback.
4. Apply the description of a simple system to the manner in which Roy describes the person.
5. Define *coping mechanisms.*
6. Describe two types of coping mechanisms.

7. Define *response.*
8. State the difference between *adaptive* and *ineffective* responses.
9. Define *adaptation level.*
10. Describe *holistic* as it relates to the human system.
11. Describe *adaptive* as it relates to the human system.

THE RECIPIENT OF NURSING CARE

Typically, nurses are viewed as caring for individuals who have become ill. However, nursing care need not focus on only one person nor need it deal exclusively with those who are sick. Consider the nurse who regularly visits the school to ensure that the children receive their immunizations. She is focusing on prevention of illness. In addition to being concerned with the health of each child, she is also dealing with the well-being of the community. Nurses are employed in industry to oversee the health of the workers. These nurses care for groups of people as well as the individual. Some nurses are involved in nursing-related research to determine more effective ways to carry out nursing activities; they are dealing with societal concerns.

Thus, the recipient of nursing care may be an individual, a family or group, a community, or society as a whole. Since the basis for any family, group, community, or society is the individual, the discussion in this text will focus on the person and the concepts involved in relating on a one-to-one basis in a nursing capacity. It should be noted, however, that in more advanced levels of nursing practice, the principles inherent in this view of the person can be applied to families, groups, communities, and society as a whole. (See Roy 1983 and 1984b.) The following discussion explores Roy's view of the person—the recipient of nursing care—as a holistic adaptive system.

THE PERSON AS A SYSTEM

In the Roy Adaptation Model for Nursing, the recipient of nursing care is viewed as a holistic adaptive system. A **system** is a set of parts connected to function as a whole for some purpose and does so by virtue of the interdependence of its parts. Consider a mercury thermometer as an example of a simple system (Fig. 2-1). The parts involved are a glass cylinder and bulb with some mechanism to indicate temperature readings, and a liquid with particular properties of expansion and contraction. By putting the liquid into the bulb and cylinder, a simple system is created for the purpose of indicating temperature. The parts are

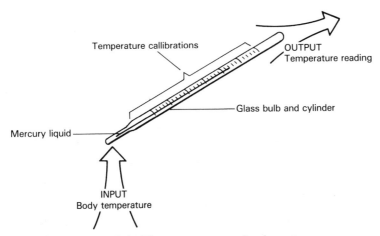

Temperature callibrations

OUTPUT
Temperature reading

Glass bulb and cylinder

Mercury liquid

INPUT
Body temperature

Figure 2-1   Thermometer as a simple system

interdependent; the bulb and cylinder would not register temperature without the liquid and the liquid would not register temperature if it were not contained in the bulb and cylinder. Neither would serve the purpose without a mechanism to indicate temperature calibration.

An example of a simple system that incorporates a feedback mechanism is an electric kettle (Fig. 2-2). Its parts (the electrical element and cord and water receptacle) serve the purpose of heating water to boiling point. In this case, the added feature of a thermostat serves to regulate the electrical input once the boiling point has been reached.

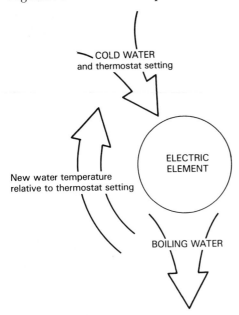

COLD WATER
and thermostat setting

ELECTRIC
ELEMENT

New water temperature
relative to thermostat setting

BOILING WATER

Figure 2-2   Electric kettle as a simple system

The electric kettle is characteristic of a type of system having four aspects: **inputs, controls, outputs,** and **feedback** (Fig. 2-3). The control mechanism is central to the functioning of this type of simple system. In the case of the electric kettle, the control detects the input (water temperature) and in turn activates a mechanism (the electrical element) to produce output (boiling water). Input consists of information being fed into the system either in respect to a standard to which the device is preset (boiling point of water) or feedback from previous output. The outputs are the actions of the system (the water boils). Information relative to the water temperature in turn serves to influence the amount of electricity fed into the system.

This description of a system can also be applied to a person. As with the typical system described previously, a living being can be described as a whole made up of parts that function as a unity for some purpose. The aspects of inputs, controls, outputs, and feedback apply in like manner.

As with a simple system, the control mechanisms are central to the functioning of a person. Roy has termed these control processes *coping mechanisms.* These coping mechanisms can be defined as innate or

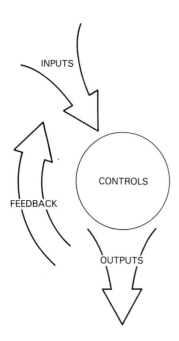

Figure 2-3 Diagrammatic representation of a simple system

acquired ways of responding to the changing environment. **Innate coping mechanisms** are genetically determined or common to a species whereas **acquired coping mechanisms** are developed through processes such as learning. An example of an innate coping mechanism in a person is manifest by shivering in response to cool temperature; an acquired or learned mechanism would be manifest by the person putting on a sweater. Coping mechanisms cannot be viewed directly; it is the output of the system or the person's response that provides an indication of coping mechanism functioning. A **response** can be defined as the behavior of the person that shows coping mechanism activity.

Inputs for the person have been termed **stimuli** and come externally from the environment (external stimuli) and internally from the self (internal stimuli). Roy defines a stimulus as that which provokes a response. Certain stimuli pool to make up another factor comprising input, the person's **adaptation level**. A person's adaptation level constantly changes. Basically, it is a changing point that represents the person's ability to respond positively in a situation. It is the limit beyond which ineffective coping behaviors are seen. According to Helson (1964), adaptation level is determined by the pooled effect of three classes of stimuli:

1. *Focal stimuli*—internal or external stimuli immediately confronting the person (e.g., a blizzard).
2. *Contextual stimuli*—all other internal or external stimuli evident in the situation (e.g., the person has no overcoat and no shelter).
3. *Residual stimuli*—stimuli that may be affecting behavior but whose effects are not validated (perhaps the person has not eaten in 24 hours).

Thus the person's ability to respond positively in a situation would be a function of the pooled effect of the three classes of stimuli identified above. The person's response is thus a function of the input stimuli and his or her adaptation level. (See Fig. 2-4.)

The individual's behavior is the output of the human system and takes the form of adaptive responses and ineffective responses. These responses are adaptive or ineffective in terms of the goals of the human system (survival, growth, reproduction, and mastery). Adaptive responses promote integrity (wholeness) in terms of these goals while ineffective responses do not contribute to these goals. These responses act as feedback or further input to the system, allowing the person to decide whether to increase or decrease efforts to cope with the stimuli.

Roy has used the terms *holistic* and *adaptive* to describe the person as a system. *Holistic* pertains to the idea that the human system

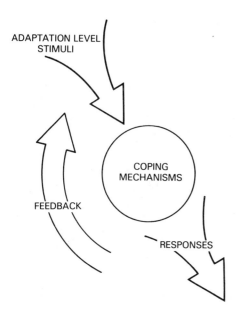

Figure 2-4 The person as a system

functions as a whole and is more than the mere sum of its parts. As will be evident as the view of the person according to the Roy Adaptation Model is explored further, all the various aspects of the person are inter-related and anything happening to one aspect will have an effect on the others.

The word *adaptive* is an integral concept in the model. *Adaptive* means that the human system has the capacity to adjust effectively to changes in the environment and, in turn, affects the environment.

The above description has provided an overview of the concepts inherent in the view of the person as a holistic adaptive system: stimuli and adaptation levels as inputs, coping mechanisms as controls, and adaptive and ineffective responses as outputs and feedback to the system.

SUMMARY

This chapter, in highlighting the major concepts of the person as viewed by the Roy Adaptation Model, has dealt with the recipient of nursing care and the person as an adaptive system. The four major as-pects of simple systems (input, controls, output, and feedback) were explored and then applied to the person when viewed as a holistic adap-tive system. The concepts of stimuli, adaptation level, response, and coping mechanisms were introduced at a beginning level. These will be explored in greater depth in the following chapters. Discussion in Chapter 3 will focus on stimuli, adaptation level, and responses, while Chapter 4 will deal with coping mechanisms and how these are observed in the adaptive modes.

EXERCISES FOR APPLICATION

1. A record player can be considered an example of a simple system. Central to its functioning are a source of power, the revolving turntable, a needle to detect the sound, and an apparatus to amplify it. Record players can normally be adjusted to accommodate several sizes of records. What aspect(s) of this system represent input, output, controls, and feedback?

2. After gardening in the hot sun for an hour, a man suddenly realizes he is thirsty. He goes over to the garden hose and turns on the tap for a drink of water. In this situation, what factor(s) could be considered stimuli? What type(s) of coping mechanisms are manifest in his behavior? What responses are observed? What is the feedback in this example?

ASSESSMENT OF UNDERSTANDING

Questions

1. Which of the following statements apply (applies) to Roy's description of *the recipient of nursing care*?
   (a) The recipient is always an individual person.
   (b) The recipient may be well or ill.
   (c) The recipient is a holistic, adaptive system.

2. Fill in the missing word.
   A _____ is a set of parts connected to function for some purpose as a whole and does so by virtue of the interdependence of its parts.

3. Identify and explain the relationships of the four aspects of the following system.
   A simple electric heating system functions to produce and maintain heat at a certain temperature. A preset point on a thermometer indicates the desired temperature while a control device (thermostat) compares the heat produced with the heat needed to reach the preset temperature and operates a switch accordingly.

4. Fill in the missing words.
   In a human system, inputs have been termed _____ _____ and _____. The controls or _____ _____ are central to function and their activity is manifest by _____ which act as feedback and further input to the system.

5. Choose the correct term from those listed below.
   _____ are innate or acquired ways of responding to
   a changing environment.
   (a) Controls
   (b) Coping mechanisms
   (c) Systems
   (d) Adaptation levels

6. State the difference between *innate* coping mechanisms and
   acquired coping mechanisms.

7. Which of the following statements applies (apply) to a *response*?
   (a) It manifests the activities of the coping mechanisms.
   (b) It is a behavior.
   (c) It is a function of input stimuli and adaptation level.
   (d) It may be innate or required.

8. Label each of the following descriptions according to whether it
   indicates an adaptive (A) or inneffective (I) response.
   (a) _____ Disrupts integrity
   (b) _____ Does not contribute to survival, growth, reproduction,
             or mastery
   (c) _____ Promotes integrity
   (d) _____ Contributes to the goals of the human system

9. Which of the following statements apply to *adaptation level*?
   (a) It is an input into the human system.
   (b) It is comprised of pooled stimuli.
   (c) It is a fixed point on the adaptation scale.
   (d) It represents a person's ability to respond positively.

10. How does the word *holistic* relate to Roy's description of the per-
    son as a system?

11. What word is used by Roy to indicate that the human system has
    the capacity to adjust to changes in the environment? _____
    _____

Feedback
 1. b, c
 2. system
    Input—The location of a preset point on the thermometer
          —Feedback that comes from the output
    Control—The thermostat that operates the switch
    Output—The heat produced
    Feedback—The environmental temperature as detected by the
    thermostat

When the thermostat detects that the environmental temperature is less than the preset temperature, it activates the switch which initiates heat production.

4. Stimuli, adaptation level, coping mechanisms, responses (or behavior)
5. b
6. Innate coping mechanisms are genetically determined or common to a species whereas acquired mechanisms are developed through processes such as learning.
7. a, b, c
8. (a) I
   (b) I
   (c) A
   (d) A
9. a, b, d
10. The human system functions as a whole; the various aspects are interrelated and anything happening to one will have an effect on the others.
11. Adaptive.

REFERENCES

Helson, Harry. *Adaptation Level Theory*. New York: Harper & Row, Publishers, 1964.

Roy, Sister Callista. "The Roy Adaptation Model of Nursing," in *Introduction to Nursing: An Adaptation Model* (2nd ed.), by Sister Callista Roy, pp. 27–44. Englewood Cliffs, N.J.: Prentice-Hall, Inc., 1984a.

Roy, Sister Callista, and Sharon Roberts. *Theory Construction in Nursing: An Adaptation Model*. Englewood Cliffs, N.J.: Prentice-Hall, Inc., 1981.

Roy, Sister Callista, "The Roy Adaptation Model: Applications in Community Nursing." in *Proceedings of the Eighth Annual Community Nursing Conference*. University of North Carolina, Chapel Hill, North Carolina, May 22, 1984(b).

_____ . "Roy Adaptation Theory (Model) of Nursing," in *Family Health: A Theoretical Approach to Nursing Care*, ed. Imelda Clements and Florence Roberts. New York: John Wiley & Sons, Inc., 1983.

Chapter 3

Stimuli, Adaptation Level, and Responses

It has been noted that the person as an adaptive system is affected by the world around and within. In the broadest sense this world is called the environment. According to the Roy Adaptation Model for Nursing, the environment is more specifically known as stimuli: focal, contextual, and residual. It is the pooling of these stimuli that make up the adaptation level, or the ability of the person to cope with the changing environment. Based on the environment and the current adaptation level, the person makes a response. The responses can be adaptive or ineffective. This chapter describes the concepts of stimuli, adaptation level, and responses.

The nurse soon learns that the person never acts in isolation, but is influenced by the environment and in turn affects the environment. Understanding this ongoing interaction and its effect on adaptation is important to nursing practice according to the Roy Adaptation Model for Nursing.

OBJECTIVES

After studying this chapter, the reader should be able to do the following:

1. Define *focal stimuli*.
2. Identify an example of a focal stimulus.
3. Define *contextual stimuli*.

4. Identify an example of the contextual stimuli related to a given focal stimulus.
5. Define *residual stimuli.*
6. Identify examples of possible residual stimuli for given focal and contextual stimuli.
7. Describe *adaptation level.*
8. Discuss the significance of adaptive responses.

STIMULI

The Roy Adaptation Model for Nursing describes three classes of stimuli that form the person's environment (Roy 1984). The naming of these stimuli and the original descriptions of how they act are based on the work of a physiological psychologist, Harry Helson (1964). However, the use of these categories by thousands of nurses has clarified their meaning within the nursing framework. Each classification of stimulus will be discussed individually and interrelations among them will be pointed out.

Focal Stimulus

The focal stimulus is the stimulus most immediately confronting the person. It is the object or event that attracts one's attention and it may be inside or outside the person. For example, a person may turn around quickly when he hears a loud noise coming from behind him, or he may feel annoyed when he hears a buzzing sound in his own head. The person focuses attention upon the stimulus and also spends energy to deal with it. Thus, in the example of internal or external noise, the person tries to find the source of the noise and to decide what to do to handle it.

With the environment constantly changing, many stimuli never become focal, that is, they never immediately confront the person. We generally do not pay attention to the weather unless it is particularly pleasant or unpleasant or is changing. Similarly, positive or negative or changing environments can become focal, or confront the person, and require a response.

As the nurse using the Roy Adaptation Model views her patient, she will note the many stimuli that may be focal for the patient. For the surgical patient, pain may be a focal stimulus, the one on which the patient focuses attention and energy. For the pediatric patient, being away from home may be the focal change. When the nurse is working in the home with the elderly patient who is recovering from a stroke, she may find that the person focuses mainly on the fear of another stroke.

Contextual Stimuli

Contextual stimuli are all other stimuli present in the situation that contribute to the effect of the focal stimulus. That is, contextual stimuli are all the environmental factors that also present to the person from within or without, but which are not the center of the person's attention and/or energy. These factors will influence how the person can deal with the focal stimulus. In our common experience with the weather, it is not the temperature alone that makes us react to the hot or cold. When high humidity is added to high temperatures the heat is less tolerable, and when a wind chill is added to cold temperatures one is more affected by the cold. While more attention is devoted to the focal stimulus, the contextual stimuli are those that also can be identified as affecting the situation.

Just as a patient may have many environmental changes that can be focal, so each of those situations can have many contextual stimuli. The person in pain may be more distressed by pain when the cause of it is unknown. Similarly, pain may be better tolerated when the person knows that it is expected and is temporary. A child may handle being away from home more easily when she can have her own toys with her and expects her parents to return. The person who fears another stroke may find that his fear is intensified by memories of his own stroke and of the death of his brother from a stroke. In these examples, we see that the contextual stimuli are also within or outside the person and that they can be positive or negative factors.

Residual Stimuli

A residual stimulus is a factor that may be affecting the person, but that cannot be validated. The person may not be aware of the influence of this factor, or it may not be clear to the observer that the factor is having an effect. For example, a person who is frightened in a storm may have forgotten that he was lost in a storm once as a child. A friend who observes that the person is very frightened may have a hunch that perhaps he had a bad experience in the past. However, in describing what is causing the fright, the observer can only consider this as a possibility since the person has never mentioned such an experience. Residual stimuli are environmental factors within or without the person whose effects in the current situation are unclear.

In looking at what is affecting the person in a given nursing situation, it is useful for the nurse to consider *possible* influencing stimuli.

In this way she can further describe the situation. For example, she may observe the child's reaction to being away from home and consider that this might be the child's first separation from her parents. The nurse frequently uses the category of residual stimuli to place her general knowledge about what influences the type of behavior observed. She then gets to know the individual well enough to decide whether that stimulus is focal, contextual, or perhaps not applicable to the patient. By using the category of residual stimuli, one has a place to include even uncertain influencing stimuli.

The nurse recognizes that focal, contextual, and residual stimuli change rapidly. The environment is changing constantly and the significance of any one stimulus is changing. What is focal at one time soon becomes contextual and what is contextual may slip far enough into the background to become residual, that is, just a possible influence. For example, when a person is watching the national weather report, he may be vaguely aware of the weather patterns in another part of the country. If he suddenly remembers that he will be travelling to that area soon, his attention focuses on what is being said. Similarly, what one had for lunch yesterday rarely has much effect on current behavior unless there was something unusual about it, such as being contaminated by bacteria. In some cases, Friday's lunch may be a focal stimulus on Saturday. Throughout this text, there are examples of the three types of stimuli and their importance in providing nursing care according to the Roy Adaptation Model.

ADAPTATION LEVEL

In Chapter 2, it was noted that the focal, contextual, and residual stimuli pool to make up the person's adaptation level. *Adaptation level* is the name given to the changing point that represents the person's ability to respond positively in a situation. Helson (1964) first used this term in a technical sense related to how the person's ability to deal with a situation comes from two aspects—the demands of the situation and the person's current internal and external resources. For example, a person responds to a storm on the basis of how severe the weather is, how important it is to travel, contingency plans for worsening weather, and perhaps fears related to a previous experience. Ability to respond positively depends upon all three types of stimuli and their current effect on the person. The focal stimulus is judged to have the greatest effect, but there may be many relevant contextual stimuli and any number of residual stimuli that can be considered. An earlier figure (Fig. 2-4) shows that the person's response is a function of the input stimuli and the person's adaptation level.

When one begins to understand the notion of adaptation level, one recognizes that the person is not passive in relation to the environment. The person and environment are in constant interaction with each other. If a person's ability to deal with a new experience is limited, one may actively seek to learn about this experience. For example, in setting up a new household, the young adult may choose to take a short course on finances. In this way, the person can change his or her own adaptation level. Similarly, one can also change the external environment. For example, if a group of employees finds that a focal concern for them is the unrealistic demands of their employer, they may take positive action together to change the employer's expectations. In this way, the person is an active participant in the process of responding positively, or adapting, to the environment. Mutual enhancement of human beings and their environment has become a social issue in the postindustrial era.

When we think of adaptation level in clinical terms, we should bear in mind that nurses meet persons who have varying levels of ability to cope with changing circumstances. These varying levels are made up of the pooled effect of the major relevant influencing stimuli. That is, at any given time the person will respond on the basis of the combined effect of the internal and external environment. As has been noted, the current internal state includes a person's past experiences, even those of which the person may not be aware. The nurse is impressed often by the extent to which persons can cope with potentially overwhelming situations. Many parents of a child with birth defects respond with love, concern, and appropriate planning. This response is related to the pooled effect of all that these persons bring to this demanding situation.

Adaptation level, then, is a concept that can be described by identifying the relevant focal, contextual, and residual stimuli in a situation. Together, these stimuli determine a range of coping for the person. Many positive life experiences may give a person a broad range of abilities to deal with life's changes. A changing situation may limit that range. For example, a single parent may have worked very hard to maintain a family and home and be an example to all her friends and colleagues. However, recognizing that she is the sole support and parent of that family, she may find it unusually difficult to handle an illness that requires even a short hospitalization.

The nurse is aware of both the strengths and limitations of the persons with whom she deals whether they are patients or co-workers. She also recognizes minor fluctuations in her own changing adaptation level in situations of fatigue and mild anxiety. Furthermore, she knows that at times the challenges of her work can tax her own resources. For example, in working with dying patients, she must call upon all her resources and sometimes those outside herself to deal with the physical and emotional demands of the situation. The nurse does not avoid these experiences, but can see them as new opportunities for growth, further extention of her inner resources, and the broadening of her adaptation range.

RESPONSES

The person as an adaptive system was discussed in Chapter 2. Recall that stimuli and adaptation level serve as input to this adaptive system and, after processing them through the regulator and cognator mechanisms, the person makes responses. These responses are called behavior. **Behavior** is defined in the broadest sense as actions and reactions under specified circumstances; it may be internal or external. A person who responds to a loud noise, by walking toward the noise is making an external response. At the same time, the person's increased heart rate is an internal response. Behaviors can be observed, measured, or subjectively reported. For example, one can see the person walk across the room, a monitor can measure heart rate, or the person may say that he feels frightened.

As the nurse views the person as an adaptive system, the output behavior shows how well the person is adapting to environmental change. This observation is key to nursing assessment and intervention. The nurse's assessment of behaviors is discussed in detail in Chapter 6.

An important concern is whether the behavior is adaptive or ineffective. In general, the judgment about the effectiveness of the behavior is made in collaboration with the person and is specific to that person and the condition and circumstances. However, the Roy Adaptation Model provides broad guidelines for judging adaptive behaviors.

Adaptive responses are those that promote the integrity of the person in terms of the goals of adaptation: survival, growth, reproduction, and mastery. To drink water when one's body fluids are depleted is an adaptive response contributing directly to survival. Similarly, to seek out new educational experiences contributes both to growth and mastery. The notion of reproduction includes the continuation of the human species by having children but it also involves the many ways that people procreate their own persons. For example, the Native American grandfather lives on in the life of his grandchild by instilling the values of the tribe in the child. One's personal contributions are propagated both through individuals and to the whole society. The cultural heritage left by poets and artists can be viewed as their own adaptive responses related to reproduction. Adaptive responses, then, promote the goals of adaptation and promote the integrity of the person. The person's adaptation has an effect upon the broader society.

Ineffective responses, on the other hand, are those that do not promote integrity nor contribute to the goals of adaptation. That is, they may, in the immediate situation or if continued over a long time, threaten the person's survival, growth, reproduction, or mastery. To refuse to eat for one day may not be a serious threat to survival, but to continue such a fast over many weeks may be a serious threat and is ineffective for survival. In judging effectiveness, then, one looks at the effect of the behavior on the general goals of adaptation. At the same time, the person's individualized goals are a major consideration. For example, there has been much discussion of the right to die. In certain stages of illness, sheer survival may not be the person's highest goal. Rather, the person may choose to be free from medical intervention to enter the final developmental stage of life, that is, death. One author (Dobratz 1984) has described this developmental stage according to the Roy model as the person's life closure. Goals of reproduction, in the sense of the legacy of self, and mastery are more prominent at this time. The total integrity of the person may be at its highest point as all of the experiences of life are brought together in this closure. Ineffective responses in this situation would be those that do not contribute to the person's own adaptive goals.

In addition to these broad guidelines for determining adaptive and ineffective responses, the nurse's understanding of the cognator and regulator mechanisms can offer further guidelines. In general, indications of adaptive difficulty can be observed in pronounced regulator activity and cognator ineffectiveness. For example, a person may have a rapid pulse and tense muscles, but may deny that anything is bothering him. The nurse recognizes that the body is automatically responding to some threat, but the person is not effectively using his cognitive and emotional processes to deal with the situation. His response of saying that nothing is bothering him is ineffective in handling the threat. Chapter 6 includes further discussion of the nurse's assessment of adaptive and ineffective behavior and how the basic concepts of the Roy Adaptation Model are used in conjunction with established norms for human behavior.

Responses, then, are the person's behavior as an adaptive system. They can be observed, measured, or subjectively reported. As the nurse helps the person promote adaptation, she must assess the person's current responses and their effectiveness.

SUMMARY

In this chapter the person's interaction with the environment has been explored. The concepts of stimuli, adaptation level, and responses have been presented. In this discussion, the specific view of environment that is put forth by the Roy Adaptation Model for Nursing has been described. Environment is viewed as internal and external stimuli which are further categorized as focal, contextual, and residual. The pooling of these stimuli determines the person's adaptation level. Based on this level, the person processes environmental changes by means of mechanisms that Roy has termed the regulator and the cognator mechanisms and then responds with adaptive or ineffective responses. These responses, in turn, affect the internal and external environment of the person. In the next chapter, the regulator and cognator mechanisms and their adaptive modes will be looked at more closely.

EXERCISES FOR APPLICATION

1. Imagine yourself in rush-hour traffic approaching an intersection at which the light for your direction of traffic has just turned to yellow. Suggest focal, contextual, and residual stimuli that might have an effect on your judgment as to what action to take.

2. From your personal experience in writing an important examination, suggest focal, contextual, and residual stimuli that serve (a) to broaden your adaptation level or range of coping abilities and (b) to limit that range.

3. In considering your own behavioral responses during the last minute, suggest two responses that can be (a) observed, (b) measured, and (c) subjectively reported.

4. Suggest two behavioral responses that would be considered adaptive in promoting your mastery of the content presented in this chapter and two that would be considered ineffective. An example of an adaptive response would be "underlining important concepts"; an ineffective response would be "daydreaming."

ASSESSMENT OF UNDERSTANDING

Questions
1. Which of the following statements apply (applies) to *focal stimulus*?
   (a) It is a factor from a person's past influencing the current situation.
   (b) It is the pooled effect of three classes of stimuli.
   (c) It is the stimulus most immediately confronting the person.
   (d) It is what is causing pain for the person.

2. What is the focal stimulus in the following situation?
   A four-year-old child is having a plaster cast changed. He has been wearing casts on his left ankle since he was six months old in order to correct a congenital problem. The second the plaster saw comes into his view, he begins to scream, calling for his mother. On previous occasions, the staff doing the procedure have had to restrain him and proceed as quickly as possible with their task.

3. Fill in the missing words.

Contextual stimuli are defined as all other _____ present in the situation that _____ to the effect of the _____ _____ stimulus.

4. In the situation described in question 2, identify three possible contextual stimuli.

(a) _____

(b) _____

(c) _____

5. Which of the following statements apply to *residual stimuli*?

(a) They require a response.

(b) They are not validated.

(c) They can be identified as affecting a situation.

(d) They are the center of the person's attention and energy.

(e) They are factors whose effects in a situation are unclear.

6. Which of the following factors could be residual stimuli affecting the child described in question 2?

(a) Absence of his mother

(b) Aversion to loud noises

(c) A previous cut from the plaster saw

(d) Lack of understanding about the procedure

(e) Observing his father being cut by a power saw

7. Which of the following statements apply to *adaptation level*?

(a) It is a changing point.

(b) It is a person's state of health.

(c) It is the person's ability to respond positively.

(d) It is the pooled effect of three types of stimuli.

8. Considering the promotion of integrity and the goals of adaptation, label each of the following behaviors as to whether it is adaptive (A) or ineffective (I).

(a) _____ Eating consistent diet of sweets

(b) _____ Using improper body mechanics while lifting a heavy object

(c) _____ Struggling while having a cast removed

(d) _____ Writing a term paper

(e) _____ Teaching a poem to a child

(f) _____ Refusing medical intervention in the final stages of a terminal illness

Feedback

1. c

2. The plaster saw

3. stimuli, contribute, focal

4. Any three of the following:
   Previous cast removal procedures
   Restraining by staff
   Absence of mother
   Noise of the saw
5. b, e
6. b, c, d, e. The situation does not provide information about these stimuli; they are not validated.
7. a, c, d
8. (a) I
   (b) I
   (c) I
   (d) A
   (e) A
   (f) A

REFERENCES

Dobratz, Marjorie Clowey. "Life Closure," in *Introduction to Nursing: An Adaptation Model* (2nd ed.), by Sister Callista Roy, pp. 497–518. Englewood Cliffs, N.J.: Prentice-Hall, Inc., 1984.

Helson, Harry. *Adaptation Level Theory*. New York: Harper & Row, Publishers, 1964.

Roy, Sister Callista. "The Roy Adaptation Model in Nursing," in *Introduction to Nursing: An Adaptation Model* (2nd ed.), by Sister Callista Roy, pp. 27–41. Englewood Cliffs, N.J.: Prentice-Hall, Inc., 1984.

Chapter 4

Coping Mechanisms
and Adaptive Modes

Coping mechanisms (innate and acquired ways of responding to a changing environment) were introduced in Chapter 2. These internal processes are broadly categorized as the regulator subsystem and the cognator subsystem.

Both cognator and regulator activity are manifested in four particular ways in the person: in behaviors indicating physiological, self concept, role, and interdependence functioning. These four ways of classifying the manifestations of regulator and cognator activity are termed adaptive modes.

This chapter focuses on the regulator and cognator subsystems as coping mechanisms; a brief description of the four adaptive modes is provided as well.

OBJECTIVES

After studying this chapter, the reader should be able to do the following:

1. State the difference between the regulator and cognator subsystems.
2. Identify specific behaviors as indicative of regulator or cognator activity.
3. Describe the processes involved in the regulator subsystem.

4. Describe the processes involved in the cognator subsystem.
5. Given an example, identify specific regulator processes involved in a situation.
6. Given an example, identify specific cognator processes involved in a situation.
7. Describe the relationship between the coping mechanisms and the four adaptive modes.
8. Differentiate among the four adaptive modes.
9. Label specific behaviors according to the related adaptive mode.

COPING MECHANISMS

In comparing the person to a typical system, Roy identified *coping mechanisms* as the controls of the human system. Coping mechanisms were defined in Chapter 2 as innate or acquired ways of responding to the changing environment.

Innate coping mechanisms are genetically determined or common to the species and are generally viewed as automatic processes; the person does not have to think about them. An example of an innate coping mechanism is a person's ability to adapt visually to changing intensity of light. When a person enters a darkened room, the iris in the eye automatically dilates to permit the entrance of more light, thus enhancing visual acuity. This response is automatic, unconscious, and innate.

Acquired coping mechanisms are developed through processes such as learning. The experiences encountered throughout life contribute to customary responses to particular stimuli. A person, as a child, soon learns an appropriate response to a ringing telephone; the ringing (stimulus) activates acquired coping mechanisms that result in a series of actions to answer the phone (response). This response is deliberate, conscious, and acquired.

Roy further categorizes these innate and acquired coping mechanisms into two major subsystems, the regulator subsystem and the cognator subsystem.

Regulator Subsystem

A basic type of adaptive process, termed by Roy the *regulator subsystem*, responds automatically through neural, chemical, and endocrine coping processes. As illustrated in Fig. 4-1, stimuli from the internal and external environment (through the senses) act as inputs to the nervous system, circulatory system, and endocrine system of the

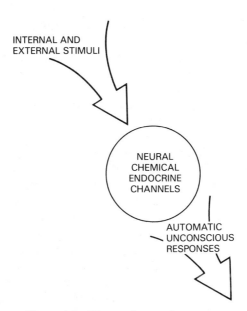

Figure 4-1   The regulator subsystem

body. The information is channelled automatically in the appropriate manner and an automatic, unconscious response is produced. At the same time, inputs to the regulator subsystem have a role in the forming of perceptions.

A mother in labor provides an example of regulator subsystem activity. During the birth process internal stimuli, both chemical and neural, initiate endocrine and central nervous system activity to produce physiological responses of labor such as uterine contraction and opening of the cervix to permit birth of the baby. External stimuli, such as medications administered during labor (for example, a drug whose action is to intensify the uterine contractions), would also affect regulator subsystem activity and, subsequently, body response.

All aspects of the regulator subsystem are so interrelated that one cannot isolate any one system as being the only active system in a particular process. As in the example above, both chemical and neural processes are involved. These complex interrelationships are further evidence of the holistic nature of the person.

Cognator Subsystem

The second major coping process is termed the *cognator subsystem*. This subsystem responds through four cognitive-emotive channels: perceptual/information processing, learning, judgment, and emotion. Perceptual/information processing includes the activities of selective attention, coding, and memory. Learning involves imitation, reinforcement, and insight whereas the judgment process encompasses such activities as problem solving and decision making. Through the person's emotions, defenses are used to seek relief from anxiety and to make affective appraisal, and attachments.

An example that illustrates all four cognitive-emotive channels is that of a person driving a car. Learning (imitation, reinforcement, and insight) is involved in mastering the skills needed to operate the vehicle. When gearshifting is required, insight as to the purpose and function of the various gear ratios and correct positioning of the gearshift is essential. The *rules of the road* and their application are handled by perceptual/ information processing and the judgment process is consistently active, although at some times it may be more effective than at others. Even the emotions are called into action, especially when another driver has suddenly to cut into the line of traffic.

As with the regulator subsystem, internal and external stimuli including psychological, social, physical, and physiological factors act as inputs to the cognator subsystem. This information is processed through the four channels mentioned previously; responses are produced. This is illustrated in Fig. 4-2.

Thinking again of our driver, the traffic light ahead of him has just turned yellow; he is already 10 minutes late for an appointment (external and internal stimuli). Through the judgment process, he decides to go through the yellow light instead of stopping. His response would probably be to step a little harder on the accelerator.

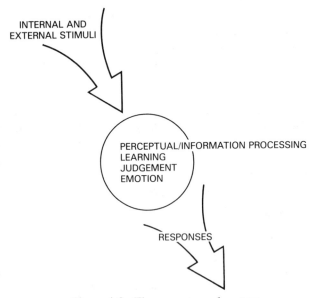

Figure 4-2   The cognator subsystem

Although the examples above have been simplified for purposes of illustration, it must be recognized that these complex relationships further illustrate the holistic nature of the person as an adaptive system.

THE ADAPTIVE MODES

Although it has been possible to identify specific processes inherent in the regulator and cognator subsystems, it is not possible to observe directly the functioning of these systems. Consider again the second example given in Chapter 2 of a simple system, the electric kettle. The purpose of this system is to heat water; the output of the system is boiling water. However, we normally cannot observe what happens in between the input to and the output from the system. The same holds true for the person as a system; we cannot observe the functioning of the coping mechanisms. Only the responses that are produced can be observed.

For this reason, Roy has identified four adaptive modes in which regulator and cognator activity are manifested. These are termed the *physiological, role function, self-concept,* and *interdependence modes* (Fig. 4-3). It is through these four major categories that responses are carried out and adaptation level can be observed. Although these four adaptive modes are discussed in greater detail in later chapters, a definition of each is provided here.

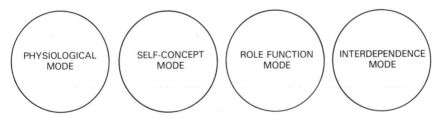

Figure 4-3   The four adaptive modes

Physiological Mode

The physiological mode as described in the Roy Adaptation Model is associated with the way the person responds physically to stimuli from the environment. Behavior in this mode is the manifestation of the physiological activities of all the cells, tissues, organs, and systems comprising the human body. As with each of the adaptive modes, stimuli activate the coping mechanisms producing adaptive and ineffective behavior. In this case, the coping mechanisms are those associated with physiological functioning and the responses produced are physiological behaviors. It is the person's physiological behavior that indicates whether the coping mechanisms are able to adapt to the stimuli affecting them.

Five needs are identified in the physiological mode relative to the basic need of **physiological integrity**: oxygenation, nutrition, elimination, activity and rest, and protection. Also inherent in a discussion of physiological adaptation are complex processes involving senses, fluids and electrolytes, neurological function, and endocrine function. These can be viewed as mediating regulatory activity and encompassing many physiological functions of the person.

Self-Concept Mode

The self-concept mode is one of three psychosocial modes; it focuses specifically on the psychological and spiritual aspects of the person. The basic need underlying the self-concept mode has been identified as **psychic integrity**—the need to know who one is so that one can be or exist with a sense of unity. Adaptation problems in this area may interfere with the person's ability to heal or to do what is necessary to maintain health. It is important for the nurse to have knowledge about the self-concept mode in order to be able to assess behaviors and stimuli influencing the person's self-concept.

Self-concept is defined as the composite of beliefs and feelings that a person holds about himself or herself at a given time. Formed from internal perceptions and perceptions of others, self-concept directs one's behavior.

The self-concept mode is viewed in the Roy Adaptation Model as having two subareas: the **physical self** (including body sensation and body image) and the **personal self** (comprised of self-consistency, self-ideal, and moral-ethical-spiritual self). The statement, "I look terrible!" is a behavioral statement related to body image; the statement, "I know I can win this game," illustrates self-ideal behavior.

Role Function Mode

The role function mode is one of two social modes and focuses on the roles the person occupies in society. A role, as the functioning unit of society, is defined as a set of expectations about how a person occupying one position behaves toward a person occupying another position. The basic need underlying the role function mode has been identified as **social integrity**—the need to know who one is in relation to others so that one can act.

A classification of roles as primary, secondary, and tertiary has been adopted for use in the Roy Adaptation Model. Associated with each role are **instrumental behaviors** and **expressive behaviors**, assessment of which provides an indication of social adaptation relative to role function. For example, associated with the role of mother are expected instrumental and expressive behaviors. Caring for the baby's physical needs would involve instrumental behaviors; holding and cuddling the baby are expressive behaviors. The manner in which the person fulfills these role expectations is an indication of role functioning.

Interdependence Mode

The interdependence mode is the second of the two social modes and focuses on interactions related to the giving and receiving of love, respect, and value. The basic need of this mode is termed **affectional adequacy**—the feeling of security in nuturing relationships.

Two specific relationships are the focus of the interdependence mode: **significant others** (persons who are most important to the individual) and **support systems** (others contributing to the meeting of interdependence needs). In relation to these specific relationships, two major areas of interdependence behavior have been identified (Randell, et al 1982): **receptive behavior** and **contributive behavior**, applying respectively to the receiving and giving of love, respect, and value in interdependent relationships. For example, a significant other for a child would be the mother. In this interdependent relationship, receptive behavior on the child's part would be allowing mother to comfort when hurt; contributive behavior would be giving Mom a big kiss upon leaving for school. The assessment of receptive and contributive behaviors provides an indication of social adaptation relative to the interdependence mode.

Each person's behavior is viewed in relation to the four adaptive modes; they provide a particular form or manifestation of cognator and regulator activity within the adaptive process. Although these modes are frequently viewed in isolation for teaching and assessment purposes, it must be remembered that they are interrelated. This is illustrated in Fig. 4-4. The four modes are depicted as four overlapping circles, central to which is a circle representing coping mechanisms. As an illustration of interrelationships, it can be noted that the physiological mode in the diagram is intersected by each of the other three modes. Behavior in the physiological mode may have an effect on or act as a stimulus for one or all of the other modes. In addition, a given stimulus may affect more than one mode or a particular behavior may be indicative of adaptation in more than one mode. Such complex relationships among modes further demonstrate the holistic nature of the person.

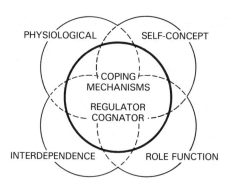

Figure 4-4 The interrelationships among modes

SUMMARY

In summary, the Roy Adaptation Model defines the person as an adaptive system with cognator and regulator coping mechanisms acting to maintain adaptation with respect to the four adaptive modes. This concept of the person is depicted in Fig. 4-5. Stimuli from the internal and external environment activate the coping mechanisms (regulator and cognator) which in turn produce behavioral responses relative to the physiological, self-concept, role function, and interdependence modes. These responses may be either adaptive and thus promote the integrity or wholeness of the person (as depicted by the arrow remaining with the adaptation circle) or ineffective and not contribute to the goals of the person (arrows extending beyond the adaptation circle).

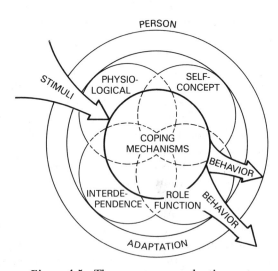

Figure 4-5 The person as an adaptive system

This visual depiction of the person as an adaptive system serves as the basis for the diagrammatic coneeptualization of the Roy Adaptation Model for Nursing used throughout this text.

EXERCISES FOR APPLICATION

1. In considering an example of a person baking bread (reading the recipe, collecting ingredients, combining them appropriately, providing suitable conditions for rising, making the loaves, and subsequently baking them), what behaviors manifest regulator and cognator activities and what processes are involved in each?
2. Identify two of your own behaviors or responses that are indicative of your functioning in each of the four adaptive modes.

ASSESSMENT OF UNDERSTANDING

Questions
1. Label each of the following descriptions of *coping mechanisms* as pertaining to the regulator subsystem (R) or the cognator subsystem (C).
   (a) _____ Respond through four cognitive-emotive channels
   (b) _____ Produce unconscious responses
   (c) _____ Involve neural, chemical, and endocrine processes
   (d) _____ Encompass perceptual/information processing
   (e) _____ Are acquired through processes such as learning
   (f) _____ Are automatic coping processes
2. Classify the underlined behaviors in the following situation as being indicative of regulator or cognator activity.

   As a young woman was driving calmly down the street, smelling fresh spring air, a small child suddenly ran out in front of her car. She slammed on the brakes and swerved to the left to avoid hitting him. As the child ran off, oblivious of the near accident, she was left in silence with the fierce pounding of her heart in her chest and her body shaking with fright.
3. Insert the appropriate words in the following description of the *regulator* subsystem.

   Stimuli from the _____ and _____ environment act as inputs to the _____ , _____ , and _____ systems of the body. Information is channelled in the appropriate manner and an _____ response is produced.

4. Match the appropriate cognator subsystem channels on the left with the activities on the right.
   1. Perceptual/Information Processing
   2. Learning
   3. Judgment
   4. Emotion

   (a) _____ Imitation
   (b) _____ Selective attention
   (c) _____ Insight
   (d) _____ Defenses
   (e) _____ Coding
   (f) _____ Memory
   (g) _____ Decision making
   (h) _____ Reinforcement
   (i) _____ Problem solving

5. In the following behaviors from the situation described in question 2, identify whether the specific regulator process involved is sensory (S), chemical (C), endocrine (E), or neurological (N). More than one process may be involved.
   (a) _____ Smelling the fresh spring air
   (b) _____ Pounding of her heart
   (c) _____ Body shaking

6. In the situation described in question 2, identify the specific cognator processes involved in the following behaviors. More than one process may be involved.
   (a) Driving down the street _____
   (b) Slammed on the brakes _____
   (c) Swerved to the left _____

7. How do the four adaptive modes relate to the coping mechanisms?

8. Label each of the following descriptions according to which one of the four adaptive models it pertains: physiological (P), self-concept (S), role function (R), or interdependence (I).
   (a) _____ Pertains to beliefs about one's self-image
   (b) _____ Pertains to love, respect, and value
   (c) _____ Formed from internal and external perceptions
   (d) _____ Pertains to biological functioning
   (e) _____ Involves sets of expectations
   (f) _____ Involves close relationships
   (g) _____ Pertains to functioning units of society

9. Label each of the following behaviors with the adaptive mode(s) it represents: physiological (P), self-concept (S), role function (R), or interdependence (I).
   (a) _____ Having one's hair set for a special event
   (b) _____ Eating three meals a day
   (c) _____ Going to work every day
   (d) _____ Studying two hours every night
   (e) _____ Attempting to lose 10 pounds

(f) _____ Congratulating a classmate on his receiving the highest
        mark in the class
(g) _____ Kissing a spouse goodbye each day before leaving for
        work
(h) _____ Drinking water on a strenuous hike

Feedback
1. (a) C
   (b) R
   (c) R
   (d) C
   (e) C
   (f) R
2. Behaviors indicative of regulator activity: pounding of her heart,
   body shaking.
   Behaviors indicative of cognator activity: driving calmly down the
   street, slammed on the brakes, swerved to the left.
3. internal, external, nervous, circulatory, endocrine, unconscious or
   automatic
4. (a) 2
   (b) 1
   (c) 2
   (d) 4
   (e) 1
   (f) 1
   (g) 3
   (h) 2
   (i) 3
5. (a) S, N
   (b) E, C
   (c) S, N
6. (a) perceptual/information processing, learning
   (b) judgment, learning, perceptual/information processing
   (c) judgment, learning, perceptual/information processing
7. The functioning of the coping mechanisms cannot be observed,
   only the responses that are produced. The adaptive modes provide
   a particular form or manifestation of regulator and cognator
   activity. Thus regulator and cognator activity relative to the four
   modes can be assessed.
8. (a) S
   (b) I
   (c) S
   (d) P

    (e) R
    (f) I
    (g) R
9. (a) S
    (b) P
    (c) R
    (d) R
    (e) S
    (f) I
    (g) I
    (h) P

REFERENCES

Buck, Marjorie H. "Self-Concept: Theory and Development," in *Introduction to Nursing: An Adaptation Model* (2nd ed.), by Sister Callista Roy, pp. 255–283. Englewood Cliffs, N.J.: Prentice-Hall, Inc., 1984.

Nuwayhid, Kathleen Anschutz. "Role Function: Theory and Development," in *Introduction to Nursing: An Adaptation Model* (2nd ed.), by Sister Callista Roy, pp. 284–305. Englewood Cliffs, N.J.: Prentice-Hall, Inc., 1984.

Randall, B., M. Tedrow, and J. VanLandingham. *Adaptation Nursing: The Roy Conceptual Model Made Practical.* St. Louis: The C. V. Mosby Company, 1982.

Roy, Sister Callista. "The Roy Adaptation Model of Nursing," in *Introduction to Nursing: An Adaptation Model* (2nd ed.), by Sister Callista Roy, pp. 27–41. Englewood Cliffs, N.J.: Prentice-Hall, Inc., 1984.

Roy, Sister Callista, and Sharon Roberts. *Theory Construction in Nursing: An Adaptation Model.* Englewood Cliffs, N.J.: Prentice-Hall, Inc., 1981.

Tedrow, Mary Poush. "Interdependence: Theory and Development," in *Introduction to Nursing: An Adaptation Model* (2nd ed.), by Sister Callista Roy, pp. 306–322. Englewood Cliffs, N.J.: Prentice-Hall, Inc., 1984.

Chapter 5

Health and the Goal of Nursing

Health and the *goal of nursing*, two closely related concepts essential to any conceptual description of nursing, were introduced briefly in Chapter 1. An understanding of the description of health as presented in the Roy Adaptation Model is contingent upon an understanding of the concepts of the *person* and the *environment* as presented in Chapters 2 and 3. Nursing acts to enhance the interaction of the person with the environment.

The concept of health as articulated in the model is in the developing stages. It is recognized that, with further consideration of the Adaptation Model from the theoretical perspective and its increasing use in practice, the clarity with which this concept can be described will be enhanced.

OBJECTIVES

After studying this chapter, the reader should be able to do the following:

1. Define *health* in terms of the Roy Adaptation Model.
2. Contrast Roy's definition of health with a general definition of health.
3. Define *goal of nursing* according to the Roy Adaptation Model.
4. Relate the concepts of *adaptation, integrity,* and *health* to the *goal of nursing.*

HEALTH

A universally accepted definition of health is that provided by the Constitution of the United Nations World Health Organization: Health is "a state of complete physical, mental, and social well-being and not merely the absence of disease or infirmity (United Nations 1968). This statement describes optimum health—a state of being. Health has also been described as a process—a continuum ranging from peak wellness to extreme poor health and death. Traditionally, health concerns were considered to be primarily physical in nature but it is becoming increasingly common to see definitions of health that encompass the more holistic perception of the person as reflected in the definition presented by the World Health Organization.

In viewing health from the nursing perspective, it is necessary to articulate a definition in terms of the related concepts of the nursing model. Recall, from Chapter 2, that the person was described as an adaptive system constantly growing and developing within a changing environment. A person's health can be described as a reflection of this interaction or adaptation. Recall, also, that successful adaptation was viewed in terms of the goals of the human system (survival, growth, reproduction, and mastery). Adaptive responses were said to promote integrity or wholeness relative to these goals—integrity implying soundness, an unimpaired condition leading to wholeness. Health can be viewed in light of the goals of the human system. The fulfillment of one's purpose in life is reflected in becoming an integrated and whole person. Thus, in the Roy Adaptation Model, health is defined as a state and a process of being and becoming an integrated and whole person. Lack of integration represents lack of health (Roy 1984).

Consider the following two situations: In the first case, a 28-year-old woman, as the result of an accident, is quadriplegic. Although confined to a wheelchair and assisted by mechanical devices, she has developed a fruitful and meaningful life as a wife, author, and painter. Her perspective on life is an encouragement to all those with whom she comes in contact.

In the second case, a 20-year-old male college student is becoming increasingly dependent on drugs to see him through his academic year. Where initially he was using them during stressful periods of examination, now he is finding that he cannot function on a day-to-day basis without their assistance. His marks are falling and he is considering withdrawing from the program.

In considering health as a reflection of adaptation with a goal of becoming an integrated and whole person, it is the first situation that exemplifies health; the woman demonstrates the integration indicative of successful adaptation while the young man is responding ineffectively to his changing environment. The need for intervention is apparent.

GOAL OF NURSING

Generally speaking, nursing's goal is to contribute to the overall goal of health care, that is, to promote the health of individuals and society. To be meaningful within the context of a nursing model, the goal of nursing must be described in terms of the related concepts of the model.

Nursing activities, as outlined briefly in Chapter 1 and discussed in depth in Part 3 of this text, involve the assessment of behavior and the stimuli that influence adaptation and intervention by managing these stimuli. Nursing acts to enhance the interaction of the person with the environment—to promote adaptation.

Consider the situation of a first-time mother hospitalized for the birth of her child. Following the birth, nursing care for the mother would be directed toward helping her adapt to her new role. In addition to physiological concerns such as nutrition, elimination, and healing, goals would relate to the mother's ability to care for the child, the support systems that she may have in place when help is required, and her psychological well-being throughout the adjustment period. In this case, the goal of nursing care is to assist the new mother in all aspects of adaptation. The nurse will identify the mother's level of adaptation and coping abilities, identify difficulties, and intervene where necessary to promote the mother's adaptation. In this manner, the integrity of the newborn child is maintained, as well. Thus, Roy defines the goal of nursing as the promotion of adaptation in each of the four modes, thereby contributing to the person's health, quality of life, and dying with dignity. It must be recognized that complete physical, mental, and social well-being (optimum health) is not possible for every person. It is the nurse's role to promote adaptation in situations of health and illness—to enhance the interaction of the person with their environment, thereby promoting health.

SUMMARY

Health is a state and a process of being and becoming an integrated and whole person. It is the reflection of adaptation—the interaction of the person and the environment. Nursing acts to promote this adaptation. The goal of nursing is stated as the promotion of adaptation in each of the four modes. In promoting adaptation, the nurse contributes to the person's health, quality of life, and dying with dignity.

EXERCISES FOR APPLICATION

1. Jot down phrases that are descriptive of your personal perception of health. Compare them to the definition of health identified in the Roy Adaptation Model.
2. List five activities that nurses perform, for example, changing surgical dressings. Is the goal of each of these activities subsumed in Roy's statement of the goal of nursing?

ASSESSMENT OF UNDERSTANDING

Questions
  1. Which of the following statements apply to the definition of *health* provided by the Roy Adaptation Model?
     (a) It is complete physical well-being.
     (b) It is a state and a process.
     (c) It is absence of disease or infirmity.
     (d) It is a continuum ranging from peak wellness to death.
     (e) It is being and becoming an integrated and whole person.
     (f) It is a state of complete physical, mental, and social well-being.
  2. *Webster's New Collegiate Dictionary* defines health as "the condition of being sound in body, mind, or spirit; especially: freedom from disease or pain." In what respect(s) is this definition different from that of the Roy Adaptation Model?
  3. Fill in the missing words.
        The goal of nursing is defined as the promotion of _____ _____ in each of the four _____, thus contributing to the person's _____, quality of _____, and _____ with dignity.
  4. The following statements relate the concepts presented in this chapter. Fill in the blanks with the appropriate concept.
        Since the _____ of nursing is to promote adaptation; and adaptation is a process of promoting _____; and _____ _____ implies soundness or an unimpaired condition leading to wholeness or unity; and the state and process of being and becoming an integrated, whole person is termed _____; then it can be stated that the goal of nursing is to promote _____.

Feedback
  1. b, e
  2. (a) Roy views health as a *state* and a *process* while *Webster's* views health as a *condition* (state).

(b) Roy views the person holistically while *Webster's* separates body, mind, and spirit and focuses on physical aspects.

(c) *Webster's* definition refers to optimum health while Roy's definition can be applied in situations of wellness and illness.

3. adaptation, modes, health, life, dying

4. goal, integrity, integrity, health, health

REFERENCES

Roy, Sister Callista. "The Roy Adaptation Model of Nursing," in *Introduction to Nursing: An Adaptation Model* (2nd ed.), by Sister Callista Roy, pp. 27–41. Englewood Cliffs, N.J.: Prentice-Hall, Inc., 1984.

United Nations. *Everyman's United Nations* (8th ed.), p. 509. New York: U.N. Office of Public Information (U.N. Publication E.67.I.2), March 1968.

Webster's New Collegiate Dictionary, Springfield, Mass.: G. & C. Merriam Company, 1980.

Part III

The Nursing Process According to the Roy Adaptation Model

Nursing is a scientific discipline that is practice-oriented. The specific activities that distinguish nursing from other disciplines are collectively termed *the nursing process*. This nursing process is a problem-solving approach for gathering data, identifying the person's needs, selecting and implementing approaches for nursing care, and evaluating outcomes of care being given.

The recipient of nursing care is the person—singly or in groups. Each person copes differently with changes in health status and it is the nurse's responsibility to help persons adapt to these changes. She must be able to identify the person's level of adaptation and coping abilities, to identify difficulties, and to intervene to promote adaptation.

The nursing process as described by Roy relates directly to the view of the person as an adaptive system. Six steps have been identified in the nursing process according to the Roy Adaptation Model:

1. Assessment of behavior
2. Assessment of stimuli
3. Nursing diagnosis
4. Goal setting
5. Intervention
6. Evaluation

The following chapters will explore each of these steps and relate it to Roy's view of the person.

It is important to recognize that, although the steps of the nursing process have been separated and specified for ease of discussion, the process is ongoing and simultaneous. For example, the nurse would be assessing the person's behaviors in one respect while she is implementing an intervention in another. This is similar to the conceptualization of the person: Although it was necessary to present each aspect as a separate entity, one must bear in mind the belief that the person functions in a holistic manner with each aspect related to and affected by the others.

Where appropriate, collaboration with the person in each step of the nursing process is important. Individuals must be involved in observation and decisions relative to their state of adaptation; they provide valuable insight that may assist the nurse in attempts to promote adaptation.

Chapter 6

Assessment of Behavior

The first step of the nursing process as described by the Roy Adaptation Model is the assessment of behavior. The goal of nursing activities is to promote adaptation. The one indicator of how a person is managing to cope with or adapt to changes in health status is behavior. Thus the first step in the nursing process involves gathering data about the person's behavior and the current state of adaptation.

Behavioral data are collected relative to each of the four adaptive modes—physiological, self-concept, role function, and interdependence—by using skills of observation, measurement, and interview. Once data have been gathered, an initial nursing judgment is made as to whether the behaviors are adaptive or ineffective. Specific and/or general criteria are provided to assist the nurse in making this tentative designation.

In this chapter, the behavior that is assessed in the first step of the nursing process is discussed. Skills involved in identifying behaviors and the criteria used in tentatively judging them as adaptive or ineffective are also presented.

OBJECTIVES

After studying this chapter, the reader should be able to do the following:

1. Define *behavior*.

2. Identify how the first step of the nursing process relates to Roy's description of the person as an adaptive system.
3. Name three skills used in behavior assessment.
4. Identify the skill used in assessing specified behaviors.
5. Given a situation, identify behaviors demonstrated.
6. Identify criteria used in judging behaviors as adaptive or ineffective.
7. Identify behaviors that demonstrate pronounced regulator activity and cognator ineffectiveness.
8. Apply criteria presented to judge specified behaviors as adaptive or ineffective.

ASSESSMENT OF BEHAVIOR

The Roy Adaptation Model views the person as a holistic, adaptive system. Input, in the form of stimuli from the internal and external environment, activates regulator and cognator coping mechanisms that act to maintain adaptation with respect to the four adaptive modes. The result is behavioral responses. These responses may be either adaptive or ineffective—the former promoting integrity of the person in terms of the goals of the human system; the latter, disrupting or not contributing to this integrity.

The person's responses are the focus of the first step of the nursing process—assessment of behavior. Figure 6-1 illustrates this step of

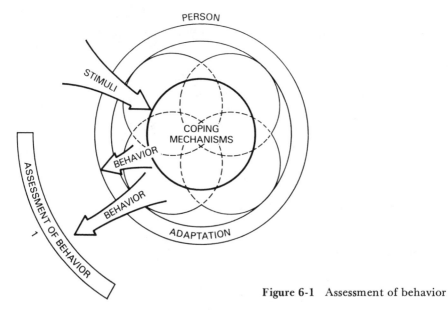

Figure 6-1   Assessment of behavior

the nursing process as it relates to the person as an adaptive system. Behavior has been defined as actions or reactions under specified circumstances. It may be observable or nonobservable. In an anxious situation, the phenomenon of "butterflies in the stomach" may occur. This is a nonobservable behavior. It must be reported or otherwise demonstrated by the person. On the other hand, observable behavior can be discerned by another. A scream by a frightened person would be an observable behavior.

Under normal circumstances, most people cope effectively with the changes that occur in their internal and external environments. However, there may be times—during an illness, for example—when there is stress placed on a person's coping abilities. The stimuli or changes being faced may be outside the person's zone of adaptation. It is often at these times that the nurse encounters the person.

In a nursing situation, the primary concern is a certain type of behavior—that which requires further adaptive response as a result of environmental changes straining the person's coping mechanisms. Important aspects of nursing are knowing how to (1) assess these behaviors, (2) compare them to specific criteria designed to assist in a judgment as to their contribution to the maintenance of integrity, and (3) identify the strengths and strains of the coping process.

In assessment of behavior, the nurse systematically looks at responses in each adaptive mode. As mentioned previously, the four adaptive modes (physiological, self-concept, role function, and interdependence) are a classification of ways of coping that manifest regulator and cognator activity. It is in relation to these four major categories that responses are carried out and that observable and nonobservable behaviors occur.

As described above, all behavior is not directly obvious to another person. Nonobservable behavior must either be reported by the person or demonstrated in some other manner. Observable behaviors typically can be seen, heard, and/or measured. Thus, in assessing behavior in each adaptive mode, the nurse uses skills of observation, measurement, and interviewing to obtain behavioral data. The scope of this text permits only a brief look at each of these methods of behavioral assessment. Proficiency in their use is achieved through knowledge and practice of the principles involved.

The nurse, when applying observational skills, uses her senses to obtain data about the person's behavior. She may see cyanotic skin color, feel a weakened pulse, smell body odor, or hear unusual chest sounds. The nurse's description of these observations would constitute behavioral data.

Behavioral responses can be measured and the values compared to preestablished normal values. The nurse may take a blood pressure reading, test a urine specimen, or have a person read an eye chart. The measured values become the behavioral data.

The nurse uses interviewing skills to listen to and purposefully question in order to obtain behavioral data. For example, a person's expression of pain should signal the nurse to ask questions regarding the nature of the pain. The person's verbal response becomes the behavioral data the nurse identifies and records.

Effective communication between the nurse and the person for whom she is caring is important in each aspect of assessment of behavior and throughout the nursing process. Without effective communication, the effectiveness of all nursing actions is questionable.

The process of data collection relative to behavior is a systematic process. In later chapters, specific behavioral data to be gathered relative to each of the adaptive modes are identified. On initial assessment, these specific data are gathered by means of skillful observation, accurate measurement, and purposeful interview. The nurse then makes an initial judgment as to whether the behavior is adaptive or ineffective. Criteria have been established to assist in this decision.

TENTATIVE JUDGMENT OF BEHAVIOR

As presented in Chapter 3, adaptive responses are those that promote the integrity or wholeness of the person in terms of the goals of the human system (survival, growth, reproduction, and mastery). Ineffective responses are those that do not contribute to these goals and thereby disrupt integrity.

A person's individualized adaptive goals are a major consideration. An example provided in Chapter 3 was that of the person in the final developmental stage—death. At this point, survival may not be the person's highest goal.

Although the parameters for the designation of adaptive responses are wide, in some areas normal values are available to guide judgment about the effectiveness of behavior. For example, charts are available suggesting normal weights and heights for specific age groups; we know normal ranges for values of pulse, blood pressure, and temperature. In other areas, expectations or generally accepted guidelines are evident. When behavior does not align with these generally accepted values, guidelines, or expectations, there is reason to suggest it may be ineffective. For example, there are expectations as to how a new mother behaves toward her baby.

In situations where *norms* are not available, Roy has hypothesized general indications of adaptation difficulty: pronounced regulator activity with cognator ineffectiveness. Some signs of pronounced regulator activity are

1. Increase in heart rate or blood pressure
2. Tension
3. Excitement
4. Loss of appetite

Signs of cognator ineffectiveness include

1. Faulty perceptual/information processing
2. Ineffective learning
3. Poor judgment
4. Inappropriate affect

Such behaviors require energy that could be used more effectively to respond to other stimuli; the responses are ineffective.

In making the initial judgment as to whether behavior is adaptive or ineffective, it is important that the nurse continually involve the person for whom she is caring. The person's perception of the effectiveness of the behavior is an integral consideration. For example, a nurse may observe that her patient slept soundly for eight hours during the night and determine that his behavior was adaptive in meeting his need for rest. However, when she asks if he feels well rested, she learns that he was actually lying quietly awake and, in fact, had slept only two hours and is feeling very tired as a result. By validating her observation with the person, the nurse changes her judgment of behavior from *adaptive* to *ineffective*. Table 6-1 highlights indicators of effective adaptation.

By initially judging behaviors as adaptive or ineffective the nurse has a basis by which to set priorities of concern. Her primary concern would be the behaviors that are disrupting the person's integrity and not promoting adaptation.

SUMMARY

The first step of the nursing process involves gathering data about the person's behavior. Through the skills of observation, measurement, and interviewing, the nurse systematically gathers data relative to adaptation in the four adaptive modes and tentatively judges the behavior as adaptive (promoting integrity of the human system) or ineffective (disrupting integrity). Criteria applied in this decision involve predetermined values, guidelines, and expectations. Where norms are not relevant, Roy's hypothesized criteria of pronounced regulator activity with cognator ineffectiveness are applied. Considering the wide parameters for adaptive responses, the person's own perception of the effectiveness of the behavior is another important factor in the decision.

In this manner, the nurse obtains an indication of whether the person is coping effectively with changes in the internal and external environment and she is able to set priorities with respect to the next level of the nursing process—assessment of stimuli.

TABLE 6-1   Indicators of Effective Adaptation

Primary Considerations

Goals of adaptation—Does behavior promote adaptation in terms of survival, growth, reproduction and mastery?

Person's own goals—What are the person's individualized goals relative to developmental stage?

Indicators

Norms—Is there departure from normal values and guidelines for expected behavior?

Coping mechanism activity—Is there evidence of pronounced regulator activity with cognator ineffectiveness?

Person's perception—Does the person realistically perceive behavior as adaptive or ineffective?

EXERCISES FOR APPLICATION

In the following situations, identify the behaviors being demonstrated and the skill used in their assessment. Label the behaviors as adaptive (A) or ineffective (I) and provide rational for your decision.

Behavior	Assessment Skills	Judgment (A) or (I)	Rationale

1. Two hours following surgery, a large amount of blood was noticed seeping through a patient's dressing. The nurse, upon taking a pulse and blood pressure, noticed that both had dropped markedly (40

and 90/60 respectively) from the readings taken the previous time. The patient who had been waking normally from his anesthetic, was now impossible to rouse.

2. A five-year-old boy was admitted to hospital accompanied by his mother. He told his nurse that he was to have an operation on his hernia and proceeded to recite all the information that he had been given on a previous "get acquainted" tour of the children's unit. He interacted readily with his new roommate until his mother announced it was time for her to leave at which point, he ran to her and began to cry.

ASSESSMENT OF UNDERSTANDING

Questions

1. Which of the following statements apply to the definition of *behavior*?
   (a) It is action under specific circumstances.
   (b) It may be observable or nonobservable.
   (c) It is readily obvious to another.
   (d) It may be adaptive or ineffective.

2. The first level of nursing assessment is primarily concerned with which of the following aspects of Roy's description of the person?
   (a) Coping mechanisms
   (b) Stimuli
   (c) Responses
   (d) Environment

3. List the three skills used by the nurse in assessment of behaviors.
   (a) _____
   (b) _____
   (c) _____

4. Label each of the following behaviors with the skill(s) most appropriate for assessing it: observation (O), measurement (M), or interview (I).
   (a) _____ Presence of sugar in a specimen of blood
   (b) _____ Fear relative to upcoming surgery
   (c) _____ Effectiveness of injection for pain
   (d) _____ Bleeding from a surgical wound
   (e) _____ Faithfulness in adhering to prescribed diet
   (f) _____ Weight loss

5. Underline the behaviors demonstrated by the child in the following situation.

   A mother noticed that her five-year-old son was not actively participating in play with other children. When she questioned him, he stated that he did not feel well and had a sore throat. The mother noticed that he appeared flushed and felt warm to her touch. Upon looking at his throat, she noticed that it was very reddened and two rather large masses of tissue were protruding from either side.

6. Which of the following statements reflect criteria used in judging whether behaviors are adaptive or ineffective?
   (a) A person states he is coping well.
   (b) Normal body temperature is 98.6°F (37°C)
   (c) Study guidelines are presented to new students.
   (d) There is pronounced regulator activity with cognator ineffectiveness.
   (e) Poor judgment is exhibited.

7. Which of the following behaviors may indicate ineffective behavior?
   (a) High blood pressure
   (b) Appropriate judgment
   (c) Ineffective learning
   (d) Normal pulse rate
   (e) Tension
   (f) Inappropriate attachments to others

8. Using the criteria presented in this chapter, label the following underlined behaviors as adaptive (A) or ineffective (I) and provide rationale for your decision.
   (a) _____ A woman of five feet weighs 60 pounds.
   (b) _____ The nurse measured her patient's blood pressure at 125/75.
   (c) _____ The patient asked the nurse three times to explain a simple procedure.
   (d) _____ A person whose pulse is 60 beats per minute states that his heart rate has been that low since he was a teenager.
   (e) _____ A person has not eaten nor had any fluid intake for two days.

Feedback
  1. a, b, d
  2. c
  3. (a) Observation
     (b) Measurement
     (c) Interview
  4. (a) M
     (b) I
     (c) I, O

(d) O

(e) O, M, I

(f) M

5. five-year-old

not actively participating in play

stated that he did not feel well and had a sore throat

appeared flushed

felt warm

(throat) very reddened

large masses of tissue were protruding

6. a, b, c, d, e

7. a, c, e, f

8. (a) I—Normally people of five feet weigh much more.

(b) A—A blood pressure reading of 125/75 is within normal limits.

(c) I—The patient appears to be demonstrating ineffective learning.

(d) A—The person confirms the behavior is normal and adaptive for him.

(e) I—Normal body requirements for fluids and nutrients are not being met.

REFERENCE

Roy, Sister Callista. "The Roy Model Nursing Process," in *Introduction to Nursing: An Adaptation Model* (2nd ed.), by Sister Callista Roy, pp. 45–51. Englewood Cliffs, N.J.: Prentice-Hall, Inc., 1984.

Chapter 7

Assessment of Stimuli

As discussed in the previous chapter, it is change in the internal and external stimuli that places stress on the person's coping abilities. The individual's behavior manifests whether or not he or she is coping effectively with these changes. The first level of assessment in the nursing process involves the assessment of this behavior and a tentative judgment as to whether it is adaptive or ineffective. The next step of the nursing process involves the identification of internal and external stimuli that are influencing the behaviors.

The skills used in assessing stimuli are the same as those used in assessing behaviors, namely, observation, measurement, and interview. Behavior manifesting disruption of integrity is of initial concern. To assist in setting priorities relative to the behavior of concern, the nurse, in collaboration with the person, identifies the focal, contextual, and residual stimuli influencing these responses. Specific contextual stimuli have been suggested by Roy and her colleagues as having an effect on behavior in each adaptive mode; these common stimuli are identified in this chapter.

OBJECTIVES

After studying this chapter, the reader should be able to do the following:

1. Define *stimuli.*

2. State the difference between the three types of stimuli.
3. Describe how *assessment of stimuli* relates to Roy's description of the person.
4. Identify six common stimuli.
5. In a given situation, identify stimuli influencing designated behaviors.
6. In a given situation, classify designated stimuli as being focal, contextual, or residual.
7. Provide an example of a behavior in one mode acting as a stimulus in another.
8. Provide an example of a focal stimulus affecting more than one adaptive mode.

ASSESSMENT OF STIMULI

For the person as an adaptive system with four adaptive modes manifesting coping mechanism activity, it is stimuli from the internal and external environment that activate regulator and cognator coping subsystems to produce either adaptive or ineffective behavior. In the first level of assessment of the nursing process, these adaptive and ineffective behavioral responses were assessed. The second level of assessment involves the assessment of the stimuli influencing these behaviors—the internal and external stimuli. Figure 7-1 illustrates this step of the nursing process as it relates to Roy's conceptualization of the person. Note the position of this second nursing activity next to the arrow designating stimuli in the conceptualization of the person.

A stimulus has been defined as that which provokes a response. Stimuli can be internal or external and include all conditions, circumstances, and influences surrounding and/or affecting the development and behavior of the person. A collective term for all internal and external stimuli is *environment*.

Stimuli are assessed relative to behavior identified in first-level assessment. Behaviors of disrupted integrity or the ineffective responses would be of initial concern. Ineffective behaviors are of concern since it is the goal of nursing to promote adaptation; the nurse wants to see that the ineffective behaviors are changed to adaptive ones. Adaptive behaviors are also important; they must be maintained and enhanced. The stimuli hold the key to the accomplishment of this goal. Changes in stimuli challenge the person's coping abilities. In many instances, stimuli can be altered by the person or the nurse, thereby enabling the person to cope more effectively. This idea will be discussed further in subsequent steps of the nursing process.

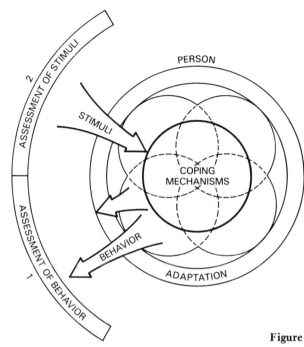

Figure 7-1 Assessment of stimuli

The skills used in assessing stimuli are the same as those used to assess behaviors—observation, measurement, and interview. As the stimuli affecting each priority behavior or set of behaviors are identified, they are classified as focal, contextual, and residual. As with step 1, and indeed each step of the nursing process, consultation with the person and validation of observations are important.

IDENTIFYING FOCAL, CONTEXTUAL, AND RESIDUAL STIMULI

The *focal stimulus* has been defined as the internal or external stimulus most immediately confronting the person. In assessing the focal stimulus, the nurse is looking for the most immediate cause of the behavior she has identified. Consider an example of a person experiencing a toothache. The focal stimulus in this situation is the fact that the person has just lost a filling from a rather deep cavity. This loss of filling and subsequent exposure of the nerve is the stimulus or change in environment with which the person is having difficulty coping.

Possible focal stimuli have been identified for given behaviors relative to each adaptive mode. These are identified in Chapters 12 through 15 where specific discussion relative to each adaptive mode is presented.

It is important to note that behavior in one adaptive mode may act as a focal stimulus in another. For example, as a manifestation of anxiety regarding her final exams, a teenage girl begins eating while she is studying and subsequently gains weight. This weight gain (physiologic behavior) may become a stimulus to the self-concept mode causing low self-esteem when she does not meet her own and other's expectations that she remain slim.

Also, one focal stimulus can affect more than one adaptive mode. The loss of a limb not only affects the physiologic mode but it may disrupt the self-concept, role function, and interdependence modes. Not only is the person's mobility affected, self-image, ability to perform roles, and interrelationships with others may be disrupted, as well.

Contextual stimuli have been defined as all other internal or external stimuli evident in the situation. They contribute to the behavior caused by the focal stimulus. For example, consider again the person with the toothache. One contextual stimulus may be that he or she has just been chewing on a very sticky piece of candy. The candy contributed to the loss of the filling but in the current situation the sugar on the exposed nerve is aggravating the pain.

Residual stimuli are the third category of stimuli influencing behavior that must be assessed. These stimuli have been defined as those having an indeterminate effect on the person's behavior; their effect has not or cannot be validated. Roy has identified two ways in which validation of a stimulus can occur: (1) The person confirms that the stimulus is affecting him; (2) the nurse has enough knowledge to establish confirmation. Residual stimuli become contextual or focal once they have been validated. When residual stimuli are identified as affecting the situation, they are no longer *possible* influencing stimuli; their effect on the person's behavior has been confirmed.

Residual stimuli affecting the person with the toothache could be the type of toothpaste being used or dental hygiene habits. If one is able to confirm that conscientious care of the teeth has not been taken, that stimulus then becomes contextual.

It is important to note that changing circumstances can change the significance of the stimuli. What is contextual at one point in time might be focal at another. For example, at the point in time when the filling was actually dislodged, the most immediate cause was the chewing of the piece of candy; this focal stimulus later became a contextual factor.

COMMON INFLUENCING STIMULI

As discussed in Chapter 3, the environment is considered to be all the internal and external stimuli affecting the development and behavior of the person. Certain contextual stimuli have been identified as having an effect on behavior in all of the adaptive modes. Table 7-1 presents an overview of these common influencing stimuli as initially identified by Martinez (1976) and selectively elaborated upon by Sato (1984).

TABLE 7-1   Common Stimuli Affecting Adaptation
Culture—Socioeconomic status, ethnicity, belief system
Family—Structure, tasks
Developmental stage—Age, sex, tasks, hereditary and genetic factors
Integrity of adaptive modes—physiological (including disease pathology), self-concept, role function, interdependence
Cognator effectiveness—Perception, knowledge, skill
Environmental considerations—Change in internal or external environment, medical management, use of drugs, alcohol, tobacco

Sato (1984) discussed culture, family, and developmental stage as of primary consideration for stimuli effecting human adaptation. Culture is described as involving socioeconomic status, ethnicity, and belief systems. Socioeconomic status provides an indication of the person's style of living and the material resources upon which the person has to draw. Different stimuli are evident in situations of different socioeconomic status. For example, an impoverished person suffering from malnutrition is affected by entirely different stimuli than those affecting a malnourished teenager from an upper middle-class family.

Ethnicity is viewed as including language, practices, philosophies, and associated values. Ethnic background may influence health practices and responses to illness. It is recognized that ethnicity is a stimulus in a person's reponse to pain. For example, Chinese people generally are more stoic when compared to the expressiveness of Italian people.

Belief system, as a component of culture, involves spiritual beliefs, practices, and philosophies and may influence all aspects of a person's life. As well as being a major support system for the person, one's belief system may have specific influence on health practices and adaptation. For example, a person's attitude toward death is affected to a great extent by the person's belief system and the extent to which these beliefs are carried into practice.

Another common influencing stimulus pertains to the family and its associated structure and tasks. Consider the different stimuli associated with a single-parent family as opposed to a nuclear or an extended family. As well, a family in the beginning stages of child rearing has different duties and responsibilities than a family whose children are grown and have left home.

Consideration of factors related to the developmental stage of the person is important in assessment of contextual stimuli affecting adaptation. Based primarily on the developmental stages and tasks identified by Erikson (1963), it is known that factors such as age, sex, and heredity influence the person's behavior, especially behavior relating to the role function mode. Further explanation of developmental stage as common stimulus is presented in Chapter 14 of this text.

The interrelationships among the aspects of the person as an adaptive system cannot be overemphasized. As noted earlier, it is important to recognize that behavior in one adaptive mode may function as a stimulus in another. Thus, lack of integrity in any area of a person's functioning (physiological, self-concept, role function, interdependence) would, in turn, act as a stimulus affecting behavior in another area. Since the nurse typically encounters persons in treatment of disease, an important consideration relative to adaptation in the physiological mode is the presence of disease pathology. This lack of integrity in the physiological mode would act as a stimulus for behavior in each of the other modes.

Another stimulus demonstrating the interrelated aspects of the person relates directly to the cognator subsystem of the coping mechanisms and involves the effectiveness with which the system is functioning. Inherent in this stimulus are the knowledge, perception, and skill possessed by the person to assist in coping with environmental stimuli. Consider an example of a malnourished individual. If the person does not recognize what nutrients constitute a balanced diet, the knowledge necessary to provide for adaptive behavior relative to nutritional health is not present and the cognator subsystem cannot perform effectively. Lack of knowledge, then, is a stimulus affecting adaptation level.

The last stimulus to be mentioned here relates to the environmental setting. Changes in environmental setting can have a pronounced effect on the person's state of adaptation. These changes tend to affect the individual's senses and include such stimuli as temperature changes, different noise levels, or unusual diet. The presence of unfamiliar people or absence of familiar ones may also be a part of environmental change. Also related to the environmental setting are drugs, alcohol and tobacco, the use of which has a distinct effect on the person's internal environment.

The effect on adaptation of each of the common stimuli identified above is a study in itself, as would be the person's effect upon environment. The discussion in this chapter is an attempt to identify common stimuli affecting a person's adaptation. It is not meant to be exhaustive; many other stimuli will be evident as each individual is assessed. The stimuli that have been described, however, include those that have been found important for primary consideration in the assessment of the stimuli affecting the individual's behavior relative to each mode.

SUMMARY

This chapter has focused on the assessment of the stimuli influencing behaviors identified during the first level of assessment. Not only are stimuli identified, they are classified as focal, contextual, or residual. A number of common stimuli were presented as affecting behavior in all individuals, their effects being manifest in each of the adaptive modes. Careful assessment of stimuli is important for later steps of the nursing process as well as for the ongoing process of assessment.

EXERCISES FOR APPLICATION

1. In thinking back over the past two hours of your own activities list five behaviors. Identify the stimulus that you consider to be the focal stimulus to each of the five behaviors.
2. A young boy has been observed and caught stealing a candy bar. What observations would you make and/or questions would you ask in attempting to determine the stimuli influencing his behavior?
3. A patient in the hospital has stated that he is unable to sleep at night. What stimuli could be contributing to this behavioral concern? List possible focal, contextual, and residual stimuli.

ASSESSMENT OF UNDERSTANDING

Questions
1. Which of the following statements pertain to the definition of *stimuli*?
   (a) They activate coping mechanisms.
   (b) They provoke responses.
   (c) They remain constant.
   (d) They may be internal or external.
   (e) They affect behavior and development.
2. Label the following descriptions as characteristic of one or more of the designated classification of stimuli: focal (F), contextual (C), or residual (R).
   (a) _____ Has not been or cannot be validated
   (b) _____ Is evident in the situation but not most important
   (c) _____ May change in significance with changing circumstances
   (d) _____ Has an indeterminate effect on the person

(e) _____ Has been validated

(f) _____ Most immediate cause of behavior

3. Describe the second level of assessment as it relates to the person as an adaptive system.

4. Which of the following are considered to be common stimuli for all individuals?
   (a) Developmental stage
   (b) Adaptation in the role function mode
   (c) Family structure
   (d) Knowledge and understanding
   (e) Ethnic background
   (f) Presence or absence of other people
   (g) Religion

5. In the following situation suggest stimuli that might be influencing the person's behavior of refusing to taste the food.

   An 80-year-old patient who had been placed on a salt-restricted diet received her first saltless meal. She announced to her nurse that she would rather go hungry than eat such tasteless food; the entire meal was left untouched.

6. In the following situation identify the stimuli that contributed to the student's performance and classify them as being focal, contextual, and residual.

   In preparation for an important exam, an anxious student who was having persistent problems in a course studied all night before the day of the test. During the writing of the exam she found that she was having trouble concentrating on the questions and remembering what she had studied. Upon handing in her paper, she commented to the instructor, "That exam was really hard; I know I didn't make a make it." She was right.

7. Suggest a behavior in one mode that could act as a stimulus in another mode.

8. Provide an example as to how the death of a child could affect behavior in each of the adaptive modes of the parents.

Feedback
   1. a, b, d, e
   2. (a) R
      (b) C
      (c) F, C, or R
      (d) R
      (e) F or C
      (f) F

3. Behavior is a manifestation of coping mechanism activity caused by the person's need to adapt to changes in the internal and external environment (stimuli). The second level of assessment involves assessment of these stimuli influencing the behaviors of concern as identified in the first level of assessment.

4. a, b, c, d, e, f, g

5. Change in normal diet
   Lack of understanding of purpose of diet
   Previous experience with saltless food
   Age

6. Had trouble concentrating and remembering—focal
   Studied all night—contextual
   Had persistent problems—contextual
   Was anxious—residual
   The exam was important—residual

7. Example: In an effort to gain acceptance by his peer group, a young boy begins taking drugs being offered him by his friend. This behavior in the interdependence mode could feasibly affect the other three modes. Drugs are known to have a detrimental physiological effect; the self-concept may manifest guilt; and the boy may be less effective in his roles (that of student, for example).

8. Physiological mode—Sleeping and eating patterns might be disrupted.
   Self-concept mode—A feeling of guilt relative to the death may be evident.
   Role function mode—Roles would be changed; the usual activities of mother or father of the child may no longer apply.
   Interdependence mode—The absence of the child may evoke feelings of loneliness.

REFERENCES

Erikson, Erik M. *Childhood and Society*. New York: W. W. Norton and Co. Inc., 1963.

Martinez. Cecilia. "Nursing Assessment Based on Roy Adaptation Model," in *Introduction to Nursing: An Adaptation Model* (1st ed.), by Sister Callista Roy, pp. 379-385. Englewood Cliffs, N.J.: Prentice-Hall, Inc., 1976.

Roy, Sister Callista. "The Roy Model Nursing Process," in *Introduction to Nursing: An Adaptation Model* (2nd ed.), by Sister Callista Roy, pp. 42-63. Englewood Cliffs, N.J.: Prentice-Hall, Inc., 1984.

Sato, Marsha Keiko. "Major Factors Influencing Adaptation," in *Introduction to Nursing: An Adaptation Model* (2nd ed.), by Sister Callista Roy, pp. 64–87. Englewood Cliffs, N.J.: Prentice-Hall, Inc., 1984.

Chapter 8

Nursing Diagnosis

Nursing diagnosis has been defined as the nurse's interpretation of assessment data (Gordon 1982) and, according to the Roy Adaptation Model, may be stated in one of three ways: (1) as a summary label for behaviors in one mode, (2) as a statement of the behaviors within one mode with the most relevant influencing stimuli, or (3) as a label that summarizes a behavioral pattern when more than one mode is being affected by the same stimuli.

Since the nursing process is a problem-solving process, once the data have been gathered the problem must be identified. This problem identification is accomplished by considering the behaviors of the person (as assessed in the first level of assessment) together with the factors causing those behaviors (as assessed in the second level of assessment) and thus establishing a nursing diagnosis. This chapter focuses on the establishment of nursing diagnoses by using the three methods identified above.

It has been found helpful, in organizing content relative to nursing diagnoses, to identify broad adaptation problems associated with each of the four modes. Roy [1984(b)] has made the following distinction between adaptation problems and nursing diagnosis: Adaptation problems are viewed as broad areas of concern related to adaptation whereas nursing diagnosis involves the judgment process and the terminology used in labeling specific instances within these broad areas of concern.

It is important to recognize that nursing knowledge relative to both adaptation problems and nursing diagnosis is in the developing stages. This chapter presents the current stage of development of nursing diagnosis as presented in the Roy Adaptation Model. Chapters 12 through 15 identify specific adaptation problems related to each of the four modes.

OBJECTIVES

After studying this chapter, the reader should be able to do the following:

1. Define *nursing diagnosis.*
2. Describe three ways to make a nursing diagnosis.
3. In a given situation, make a nursing diagnosis using each of the three methods.
4. Prioritize given nursing diagnoses according to the hierarchy of goals of the human system.

MAKING A NURSING DIAGNOSIS

Data collected thus far in the nursing process take the form of statements about the person's behavior that has been observed, measured, or subjectively reported and statements about the focal, contextual, and residual stimuli that are or may be influencing these behaviors. The third step of the nursing process involves the formulation of statements that interpret these data. Such a statement is the nursing diagnosis and is depicted in the diagrammatic representation of the Roy Adaptation Model in Fig. 8-1. The nursing diagnosis is a statement about the person. Roy has described three ways of establishing a nursing diagnosis from the data gathered in the first and second levels of assessment.

In the first method, assessment information is clustered and labeled according to a suggested typology related to each of the four adaptive modes. A typology of common adaptation problems that has evolved throughout the development and refinement of the Roy Adaptation Model is presented in Table 8-1. This typology represents commonly recurring adaptation problems.

Consider the assessment data associated with the physiologic adaptation problem of shock. Certain behaviors are characteristic of all types of shock. For example, pulse is rapid and thready, breathing is rapid and shallow, blood pressure tends to rise at first and then fall. The person feels clammy and looks pale and may be agitated or confused.

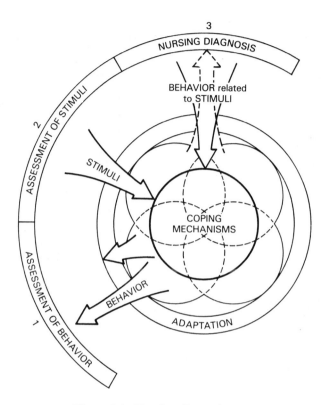

Figure 8-1 Nursing diagnosis

All these behaviors are indicative of inadequate circulation and thus insufficient oxygenation of body tissue.

Shock can result from a variety of causes (stimuli): loss of blood volume, an infectious process in the body, or a stressful physical or emotional event to name but a few.

The above-mentioned assessment information can be clustered and labelled "shock." Shock is a common adaptation problem of the physiologic mode and the person's need for oxygenation.

The second method described by Roy [1984(a)] for making a nursing diagnosis involves stating the behavior together with the most relevant stimuli. As in the first method, behaviors and stimuli can be clustered within each adaptive mode with the most relevant stimuli. Advantages of this method are twofold: (1) It allows for the incompleteness of the typology of problems; and (2) it provides more specific indications for nursing intervention since, as will be seen in Chapter 10, nursing interventions relate directly to stimuli.

Consider again the person demonstrating the symptoms associated with shock. An example of a nursing diagnosis using the second method

---

TABLE 8-1   Working Typology of Common Adaptation Problems (Revised)

A. **Physiological Mode**
   1. *Oxygenation*
      Hypoxia
      Shock
      Overload
   2. *Nutrition*
      Malnutrition
      Nausea
      Vomiting
   3. *Elimination*
      Constipation
      Diarrhea
      Flatulence
      Incontinence
      Urinary retention
   4. *Activity and Rest*
      Inadequate physical activity
      Potential disuse consequences
      Inadequate rest
      Insomnia
      Sleep deprivation
      Excessive rest
   5. *Skin Integrity*
      Itching
      Dry skin
      Pressure sores

B. **Self-Concept Mode**
   1. *Physical Self*
      Decreased sexual self-concept
      Aggressive sexual behavior
      Loss
   2. *Personal Self*
      Anxiety
      Powerlessness
      Guilt
      Low self-esteem

C. **Role Function Mode**
      Role transition
      Role distance
      Role conflict
      Role failure

D. **Interdependence Mode**
      Separation anxiety
      Loneliness

Source: Sister Callista Roy, *Introduction to Nursing: An Adaptation Model* (Englewood Cliffs, N.J.: Prentice-Hall, Inc., 1984) p. 56.

---

could be "rapid, thready pulse resulting from blood loss" or, by clustering the assessed behaviors as illustrated in the first method, "symptoms of shock resulting from injury received in motor vehicle accident." "Symptoms of shock" represents the clustered behaviors. As with method 1, the nursing diagnosis relates specifically to the physiological mode.

The third method of making a nursing diagnosis provides for the fact that one simulus may cause behaviors in more than one mode. An example used previously was that of a person suffering the loss of a limb. Assessment data could include behaviors indicative of lowered self-esteem resulting from changes in body image, difficulties in role performance, changes in dependence requirements, in addition to associated physiologic adaptation problems such as loss of appetite and disturbed sleep patterns. A nursing diagnosis that recognizes the interrelatedness of these data and crosses modes would be "depression related to the loss of limb."

The advantage of the third approach to nursing diagnosis, that of summarizing behaviors in more than one mode being affected by the same stimulus, is that the holistic functioning of the person and the interrelatedness of modes are recognized.

Nursing diagnoses may pertain to both adaptive and ineffective situations. Examples of positive diagnoses are given in later chapters. As with the first two levels of assessment, setting priorities is inherent in the third step of the nursing process. Once nursing diagnoses have been formulated, they are prioritized according to their urgency relative to the hierarchy of goals of the human system, namely, survival, growth, reproduction, and mastery. A nursing diagnosis of a life-threatening situation would be of primary importance.

Where appropriate, collaboration with the person when formulating nursing diagnoses and establishing priorities is invaluable. It is not only important that individuals are actively involved in observations and decisions relative to their state of adaptation, they often provide valuable insight that may assist the nurse in efforts to promote adaptation.

SUMMARY

Nursing diagnosis as the third step of the nursing process involves the interpretation of data collected relative to the behaviors of the person and the stimuli influencing these behaviors. Roy has identified three methods of making nursing diagnoses including summary labels pertaining to one mode, statements of behaviors and relevant stimuli pertaining to one mode, and summary labels for behaviors in several modes being affected by the same stimuli.

Priority setting is inherent in this step of the nursing process as it was in steps 1 and 2.

EXERCISES FOR APPLICATION

1. Formulate a nursing diagnosis relative to the following situation.

   A child is complaining of severe stomach cramps and has had six loose bowel movements within two hours. Upon investigation it is discovered that he had eaten three green apples from the neighbor's crabapple tree.

2. A common physiological adaptation problem identified in the nursing diagnosis typology is "malnutrition." Suggest assessment data

(behaviors and stimuli) that could be clustered and labelled with a nursing diagnosis of "malnutrition."

3. "Substance abuse" is identified in the Roy Adaptation Model as a nursing diagnosis that crosses all modes. Suggest assessment data in each of the modes that could be incorporated into a nursing diagnosis of "substance abuse."

ASSESSMENT OF UNDERSTANDING

Questions

1. Which of the following statements pertain to the definition of *nursing diagnosis*?
   (a) It is a statement relating behaviors and stimuli.
   (b) It may encompass several modes.
   (c) It is a description of physiological problems.
   (d) It is the interpretation of assessment data.
   (e) It is equivalent to a problem statement.
   (f) It is concerned with adaptive and ineffective situations.
   (g) It involves the specification of a disease process.

2. The descriptions on the right pertain to the methods of making a nursing diagnosis listed on the left. Label each description according to the method(s) to which it pertains.

   1. Summary label for one mode
   2. Statement of behaviors and stimuli for one mode
   3. Summary label for behaviors in more than one mode being affected by same stimuli

   (a) _____ Provides specific indications for nursing intervention.
   (b) _____ Typology is used for labeling clustered assessment information.
   (c) _____ Allows for incompleteness of typology of problems.
   (d) _____ Useful method for identifying common adaptation problems.
   (e) _____ Assessment data for one mode are clustered and labelled.
   (f) _____ Recognizes the interrelatedness of modes.
   (g) _____ Provides for the fact that one stimulus may affect several modes.

3. Using each of the three methods of making a nursing diagnosis presented in this chapter, formulate a nursing diagnosis statement relative to the behaviors and stimuli underlined in the situation below. Your statements need not include all behaviors and stimuli.

   A 55-year-old woman has <u>lost the use of the right side</u> of her body as a <u>result of a stroke</u>. She is presently in a program of rehabilitation which is aimed at helping her achieve a degree of independence relative to her activities of daily living. She <u>appears to lack enthusiasm</u> for the program and <u>states that she can see no reason to make an effort</u> to become active again as she <u>has lost her position</u> as an executive secretary. Since <u>she lives alone</u>, she <u>feels she could not manage</u> on her own anyway. She <u>states she is just not motivated</u> to participate.

4. The following statements are examples of nursing diagnoses related to one person who was brought to an emergency department. Prioritize them in order of importance as they relate to the hierarchy of goals of the human system ("1" is top priority).

   (a) _____ Absence of support system since family are not aware of accident

   (b) _____ Altered mobility as a result of a fractured ankle

   (c) _____ Inability to jog three miles of day due to skiing injury

   (d) _____ Deteriorating symptoms of shock due to accident

Feedback

1. a, b, d, e, f
2. (a) 2
   (b) 1
   (c) 2
   (d) 1
   (e) 1
   (f) 3
   (g) 3
3. Method 1: "Loss"—The woman has lost the use of the right side of her body due to a stroke. She can no longer physically perform her job nor can she care for herself. "Loss" is a common problem associated with the physical self-concept.

   Method 2: "Loss of use of right side of body as a result of a stroke"—A statement of behavior is connected to the relevant stimulus.

   Method 3: "Depression as a result of a stroke"—Both the self-concept and interdependence modes are affected.

"Depression" provides a summary label for the behaviors evident in each mode.

4. (a) 3
   (b) 2
   (c) 4
   (d) 1

REFERENCES

Gordon, Marjory. *Nursing Diagnosis: Process and Application.* New York: McGraw-Hill Book Co., 1982.

Roy, Sister Callista. "The Roy Model Nursing Process," in *Introduction to Nursing: An Adaptation Model* (2nd ed.), by Sister Callista Roy, pp. 42–63. Englewood Cliffs, N.J.: Prentice-Hall, Inc., 1984a.

——. "Adaptation in the Physiological Mode," in *Introduction to Nursing: An Adaptation Model* (2nd ed.), by Sister Callista Roy, pp. 89–90. Englewood Cliffs, N.J.: Prentice-Hall, Inc., 1984b.

Chapter 9

Goal Setting

Once the nurse has assessed the person's behavior and the stimuli influencing that behavior and has formulated nursing diagnoses from the assessment information, she then must establish goals. Goal setting has been defined as the establishment of clear statements of the behavioral outcomes of nursing care for the person (Roy 1984). This chapter will describe goal setting as it is related to the other steps of the nursing process.

OBJECTIVES

After studying this chapter, the reader should be able to do the following:

1. Define *goal setting*.
2. State the difference between short-term and long-term goals.
3. In given goal statements, identify the behavior to be observed, the change expected, and the time frame involved.
4. Derive complete goal statements when provided with assessment data and nursing diagnoses.

ESTABLISHING GOALS

The general goal of nursing intervention has been defined previously as to maintain and enhance adaptive behavior and to change ineffective behavior to adaptive. The person's behavior is the focus of this general statement and likewise, when establishing specific goals, the person's behavior is the focus.

Throughout the first and second levels of assessment, the person's behavior and the stimuli influencing it have been identified and recorded. This information was then formulated into nursing diagnoses. Step 4 of the nursing process, goal setting, involves the statement of behavioral outcomes of nursing care that will promote adaptation. Figure 9-1 illustrates goal setting as it relates to the other steps of the nursing process.

Recall from Chapter 6 the person who, following surgery, was demonstrating a progressive drop in blood pressure due to hemorrhage from his incision. A nursing diagnosis could be worded, "Blood pressure 90/40 related to hemorrhage." A goal for this person could be stated as follows: "The patient's blood pressure measurement will stabilize in

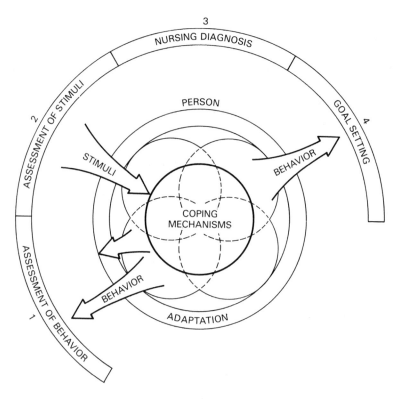

Figure 9-1 Goal setting

a range of 110/70–130/80 within 30 minutes." This is a short-term goal that identifies a behavioral outcome promoting adaptation.

Goals may also be long term. A long-term goal pertaining to the example may be, "The patient will be able to return to his job on a part-time basis within six weeks."

The designation of goals as long or short term is relative to the situation involved. For some problems, especially those that are life threatening, short-term goals may be formulated on a minute-to-minute basis; long-term goals on a day-to-day basis. In other situations, in the psychosocial realm, for example, short-term goals may involve the time frame of a week; long-term goals, months.

A goal statement should designate not only the behavior to be observed but the manner in which the behavior will change (as observed, measured or subjectively reported), and the time frame in which the goal is to be attained. Consider the following:

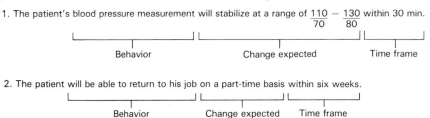

1. The patient's blood pressure measurement will stabilize at a range of $\frac{110}{70} - \frac{130}{80}$ within 30 min.

    Behavior   Change expected   Time frame

2. The patient will be able to return to his job on a part-time basis within six weeks.

    Behavior   Change expected   Time frame

Notice how each of the goals demonstrates the three elements identified above. These elements are important in the evaluation of goal attainment.

In these examples, the goals focus on ineffective behaviors in an attempt to change them to adaptive behaviors. However, it may be just as important to focus on adaptive behaviors in an effort to maintain and enhance them. Consider the following situation: A five-year-old boy, newly admitted to hospital for surgery, was interacting readily with his new roommate until it was time for his mother to leave, at which point, he began crying and clinging to her hand. In this situation, the goal might focus on the adaptive behavior of interaction with roommate. The goal might be, "Within five minutes of mother's departure, child will be playing happily with roommate as evidenced by participation in mutual activity."

Where possible, the person should be actively involved in the formulation of behavioral goals. This involvement provides the nurse with the opportunity to explain rationale behind certain goals and gives the person the chance to suggest goals and evaluate whether others are realistic. As well, a person who is actively involved in the formulation of goals is more likely to be committed to their attainment. Consider the following goal: "Within 12 hours after surgery, the patient will stand unsupported by the bed for five minutes." Generally, it is considered important for persons undergoing surgery to be mobile as soon as possible following return from the operating room. The person involved in the formulation of this goal and who understands the underlying rationale is more likely to strive to achieve it than someone who hears for the first time in pain and drowsiness, "It's time to get you out of bed."

SUMMARY

The general goal of nursing intervention is to promote adaptation by maintaining and enhancing adaptive behavior and changing ineffective behavior to adaptive. Thus, the specific goals of nursing intervention are stated in terms of the resulting adaptive behaviors expected of the person. Goals may be either short term or long term but must identify specific behaviors to be demonstrated by the person as well as the time frame and the manner in which the behavior would change. As with each previous step of the nursing process, the person should be involved when possible in the formulation of these goals.

EXERCISES FOR APPLICATION

1. Formulate three goals for yourself ensuring that each contains the three elements identified in this chapter.
2. Suggest a behavioral goal that could apply to you as the reader of this book upon your completion of this chapter. It should apply to the knowledge gained from reading the chapter.

ASSESSMENT OF UNDERSTANDING

Questions
1. Which of the following statements apply to *goal setting* as the fourth step of the nursing process?
   (a) Adaptive and ineffective behaviors may be involved.
   (b) It is necessary to know how attainment of the goal will be demonstrated.
   (c) The person's behavior is the focus.
   (d) A time frame must be included.
   (e) Statements describing behavioral outcomes are formulated.
2. Label the following goal statements as short term (S) or long term (L).

(a) _____ The patient's blood pressure will return to 120/80 within 15 minutes.

(b) _____ The patient will sleep tonight as evidenced in the morning by statements that he slept well and feels rested.

(c) _____ The patient will lose 20 pounds by the time she is weighed at her next appointment in three months.

(d) _____ The patient will demonstrate an understanding of insulin calculations by calculating his own dosage beginning tomorrow morning.

(e) _____ The patient will regain use of his hand within four weeks as demonstrated by a full range of motion.

3. For two of the goal statements in question 2, identify the behaviors, change expected, and time frame involved.

Behavior	Change Expected	Time Frame

4. Formulate several goal statements for each of the following segments of assessment information and nursing diagnoses.

Behavior	Stimuli	Nursing Diagnosis
(a) 16-year-old girl. Weighs 85 pounds. Height 5 feet 7 inches. States she does not eat breakfast and has only candy bars for lunch. Feels tired. Appears drawn and pale.	Inadequate caloric and nutritive intake. Always short of time in morning. Peer group does not eat lunch. Parents work; must prepare meals herself. Does not understand principles of good nutrition.	Malnutrition
(b) Elderly male patient. Withdrawn. Uncommunicative. Refuses to do anything for himself. States "No one cares whether I'm dead or alive." States "I'll never leave this place."	Long-term hospitalization. Hospital is long distance from home and family. Has one close relative (a son) who can visit only occasionally.	Loneliness

Feedback
1. a, b, c, d, e
2. (a) S
   (b) S
   (c) L
   (d) S
   (e) L
3.

Behavior to Observe	Change Expected	Time Frame
(a) Blood pressure	Blood pressure returns to 120/80.	Within 24 hours
(b) Sleep	He slept well and feels rested.	Tonight
(c) Weight	Lose 20 pounds.	In 3 months
(d) Understanding of insulin	Calculates own dosage.	Each morning
(e) Use of hand	Full range of motion.	Within 4 weeks

4. (a) Patient will begin to gain weight as evidenced by a measured gain of five pounds in one month.
   Patient will eat regular nutritious meals within one week as evidenced by a daily diary of food intake.
   Patient's appearance will improve within six months as evidenced by weight gain and improved coloring.
   Patient will have more energy within one week as evidenced by her statements that she feels less tired and has more energy.
   (b) The patient will begin to interact with other patients and staff by becoming actively involved in an occupational therapy session on a daily basis beginning tomorrow.
   Within two days, the patient will begin to assume responsibility for several self-care tasks as demonstrated by shaving himself and cleaning his own false teeth.
   Within two weeks, the patient will begin to demonstrate optimism for the future by inquiring about potential for discharge to alternative care agency.

REFERENCE

Roy, Sister Callista. "The Roy Model Nursing Process," in *Introduction to Nursing: An Adaptation Model* (2nd ed.), by Sister Callista Roy, pp. 42–63. Englewood Cliffs, N.J.: Prentice-Hall, Inc., 1984.

Chapter 10

Intervention

Once the goals have been established relative to behaviors that will promote adaptation, the nurse must determine how she can intervene to assist the person in attaining these goals. This is the fifth step in the nursing process.

Intervention involves the selection and implementation of approaches and is based directly on the view of the person as an adaptive system. The person's ability to adapt or respond positively to a change taking place depends on (1) the degree of change taking place (focal stimulus), and (2) the state of the person dealing with the change (adaptation level).

In order to promote adaptation, it may be necessary to change the focal stimulus or to broaden the adaptation level by managing other stimuli present. Management of stimuli may involve altering, increasing, decreasing, removing, or maintaining stimuli. In selecting approaches, the nurse considers possible alternatives and then selects the approach with the highest possibility of obtaining the desired results. Intervention always involves the management of stimuli.

The major concepts presented in this chapter are thus intervention as the management of stimuli, identification of possible approaches, and subsequent analysis, selection, and implementation of the selected approaches.

OBJECTIVES

After studying this chapter, the student should be able to do the following:

1. Describe *intervention* as the fifth step of the nursing process.
2. Explain the relationship of nursing intervention to Roy's view of the person.
3. Given a simple nursing diagnosis, establish several possible approaches to nursing intervention.
4. In a given situation, suggest the consequences of each approach and their probability of occurrence.
5. In a given situation, select the nursing intervention with the highest probability of success.
6. In a given situation, identify actions that could serve to alter appropriately a specific stimulus.

INTERVENTION AS THE MANAGEMENT OF STIMULI

In Roy's description of the person as an adaptive system, stimuli from the internal and external environment activate the coping mechanisms to produce behaviors. When ineffective behavior is identified, there is evidence that the coping mechanisms are not able to adapt effectively to the stimuli affecting them. The first three steps of the nursing process involve the assessment of these behaviors and the stimuli causing them and the amalgamation of this information into the nursing diagnosis. Subsequent goal setting is the statement of the desired behavioral outcomes of nursing care relative to the problem areas identified. Intervention focuses on the manner in which these goals are to be attained. Just as the focus of goal setting is the person's behavior, the focus of intervention is the stimuli causing the behavior. Figure 10-1 demonstrates this in terms of the Roy Adaptation Model.

As was identified in Chapter 2, the person's ability to adapt or respond positively to a change taking place depends upon the focal stimulus and the adaptation level. The focal stimulus is the degree of change taking place; adaptation level is a changing point determined by the pooled effect of the three classes of stimuli and represents the person's ability to respond positively in a situation. In order to promote adaptation, it may be necessary to manage other stimuli present. Management of stimuli involves altering, increasing, decreasing, removing, or maintaining them. Altering the stimuli enhances the ability

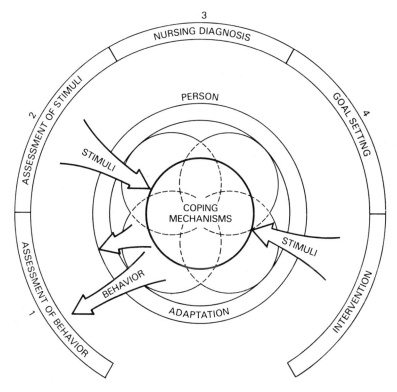

Figure 10-1 Intervention

of the person's coping mechanisms to respond positively; the result is adaptive behavior.

IDENTIFICATION AND ANALYSIS OF POSSIBLE APPROACHES

The identification of possible approaches to nursing intervention involves the selection of which stimuli to change. Roy incorporates the nursing judgment method as presented by McDonald and Harms (1966) in her description of this sixth step of the nursing process. In this method, possible approaches are listed and the approach with the highest probability of attaining the goal is selected. In applying this method to the Roy Model, the stimuli affecting a specific behavior are listed; then the consequences of changing each stimulus are identified together with the probability of their occurrence. The value of the consequence is then judged as *desirable* or *undesirable*. This is done in collaboration with the person, when appropriate.

Consider an example of the person who is unable to sleep in the hospital environment. Second-level assessment yielded the following stimuli as contributing to this sleeplessness:

> Noise level (focal)
> Uncomfortable bed (contextual)
> Person is hungry (contextual)

Application of the Nursing Judgment Method to these factors is provided in Table 10-1.

TABLE 10-1   The Nursing Judgment Method as Applied to Selection of Approaches

Alternative Approach	Consequence	Probability	Value
Alter noise level	Enhance sleep	High	Desirable
	Not enhance sleep	Low	Undesirable
Alter comfort of bed	Enhance sleep	High	Desirable
	Not enhance sleep	Low	Undesirable
	Disrupt intravenous	Low	Undesirable
Alter hunger	Enhance sleep	Moderate	Desirable
	Not enhance sleep	Moderate	Undesirable
	Disrupt plans for surgery in morning	High	Undesirable

The first approach, that of altering the stimulus of noise level, has the best probability of accomplishing the desired goal with undesirable consequences having a low probability. On the other hand, the third approach does not have a high probability of achieving the desired result and the undesirable consequence of disrupting plans for surgery is highly probable.

Whenever possible, the focal stimulus should be the focus of nursing interventions but, when this is not possible, contextual stimuli must be managed in an effort to broaden adaptation level. It may also be appropriate to use several approaches in combination. For example, a person may be suffering severe pain due to the focal stimulus of a terminal disease process. In this case, it is not possible to deal with the disease itself; efforts must be directed towards contextual factors enabling the person to cope with the disease. A personal support system may be one of the stimuli that must be increased or maintained.

IMPLEMENTATION OF SELECTED APPROACH

Once the most appropriate approach to nursing intervention has been selected, the nurse must determine and initiate the steps that will serve to alter the stimulus appropriately. Having decided that altering the noise level is the best approach to the patient's sleeplessness, she must determine how to do it. Shutting the door to the person's room might help; it may be possible to reduce the volume of the paging system. It may be necessary to move the person away from a disruptive roommate.

Having accomplished the nursing intervention, the nurse then proceeds to evaluate its effectiveness, as discussed in the following chapter.

SUMMARY

Nursing intervention as the selection and implementation of approaches focuses on the management of stimuli affecting behaviors of concern. Each stimulus is judged relative to the consequence of its alteration. The stimuli that are changed are those with the greatest probability of producing desirable results in terms of the identified goals.

EXERCISES FOR APPLICATION

1. Imagine yourself as a student who has just received a failing grade on an examination. Suggest several stimuli (focal, contextual), that may have influenced the poor performance. Identify and analyze possible approaches to the problem relative to the stimuli. Use the following table as a guideline. Select the approach with the highest probability of success.

Alternative Approach	Consequence	Probability	Value

2. The following table represents a segment of information obtained from steps 1 to 4 of the nursing process relative to an 80-year-old male patient hospitalized for a fractured hip. Following surgical insertion of a pin and plate, there is a need to increase his mobility. Continue with step 5 of the nursing process and select interventions that would assist in the achievement of the specified goals.

Behavior	Stimuli	Nursing Diagnosis	Goals
Appears apprehensive. States "I'm afraid. I can't possibly support myself; I'm too weak."	Pain increases when he tries to move (focal). Has not been eating well (contextual). Lack of understanding of postoperative routine.	Apprehensive due to lack of understanding and pain.	Patient will demonstrate increased confidence in his ability to move by attempting to get out of bed with assistance in ½ hour.
States he is having pain.	Trauma from fracture and subsequent surgery.	Pain due to injury.	Patient will experience relief from pain in 15 minutes as evidenced by statement of same.
Appears uncooperative. Asks "Why do I have to move anyway?"	Lack of understanding of importance of mobility.	Uncooperative due to lack of understanding.	Patient will cooperate with attempts to increase his mobility by following instructions the next time he is asked to try to get up.

ASSESSMENT OF UNDERSTANDING

Questions
1. Which of the following statements apply to *intervention*, the fifth step of the nursing process?
   (a) It is directed ideally towards the focal stimulus.

(b) It involves management of behavior.
(c) It may involve broadening the adaptation level.
(d) It focuses on establishing behavioral goals.
(e) It deals directly with the coping mechanisms.
(f) It involves the use of all possible approaches.
(g) It aims to enhance adaptive behavior.

2. Intervention as the fifth step of the nursing process is directly related to Roy's view of the person as an adaptive system. In the
following diagram several aspects of the Roy model are identified
by a number. For each number, write a descriptive statement ex-
plaining the relationship of the aspect identified to intervention.

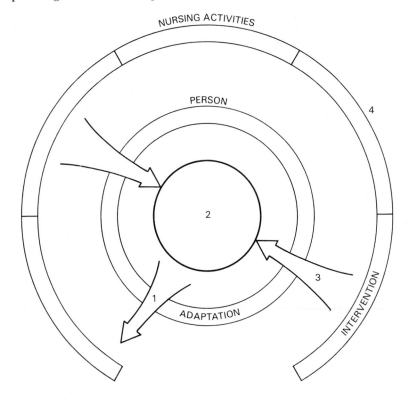

3. In the *Assessment of Understanding* section of Chapter 9, an example of a teenager suffering from malnutrition was provided. Some
of that situation is reviewed below:

Behavior	Stimuli	Nursing Diagnosis

16-year-old girl
Weight 85 pounds
Height 5 feet 7 inches
States she does not
  eat breakfast and
  has only candy
  bars for lunch
Feels tired
Appears drawn and
  pale
	Inadequate caloric and
	  nutritive intake (focal)
	Does not understand
	  principles of good
	  nutrition (contextual)
	Must prepare meals her-
	  self (contextual)
		Malnutrition

One goal was identified as, "Patient will eat regular nutritious meals within one week as evidenced by a diary of food intake." Establish three possible approaches to nursing intervention based on the assessment data provided above. Use column I of the table provided below.

I	II	III	IV
Alternative Approach	Consequences	Probability	Value

4. For each of the alternative approaches suggested for the situation in question 3, suggest consequences and the probability and value of occurrence. Use columns II, III, and IV of the table provided above.

5. Based on the information derived in questions 3 and 4, select the approach with the highest probability of success.

6. Assuming that the person in the above situation is hospitalized, list three actions that would serve to alter the stimulus identified in question 5.

    (a) _____

    (b) _____

    (c) _____

Feedback

1. a, c, g
2. 1—Behavior: Intervention is directed to the ultimate goal of changing ineffective behaviors to adaptive and maintaining adaptive
   behaviors.
   2—Coping mechanism: When ineffective behavior is evident, coping
   mechanisms are not able to cope effectively with stimuli affecting them; intervention is aimed at enhancing a person's coping
   abilities.
   3—Stimuli: Intervention involves the management of stimuli.
   4—Goal Setting: Goal setting provides the basis for intervention by
   describing desired behavioral outcomes.
3. & 4.

I	II	III	IV
Alternative Approach	Consequence	Probability	Value
Alter caloric and nutritive intake	Enhance nutritional status	High	Desirable
	Not enhance nutritional status	Low	Undesirable
Alter understanding of principles of good nutrition	Enhance nutritional status	High	Desirable
	Not enhance nutritional status	Low	Undesirable
	Create information overload	Low	Undesirable
Alter situation of meal preparation	Enhance nutritional status	High	Desirable
	Not enhance nutritional status	Low	Undesirable
	Lead to overeating	Moderate	Undesirable

5. Alter caloric and nutritive intake
6. (a) Investigate possibility of a special diet
   (b) Encourage frequent intake of food
   (c) Teach importance of good nutrition (this incorporates the
   second alternative approach)

REFERENCES

McDonald, F. J., and Mary Harms. "Theoretical Model for an Experimental Curriculum," *Nursing Outlook*, 14, no. 8 (August 1966): 48–51.

Roy, Sister Callista. "The Roy Model Nursing Process," in *Introduction to Nursing: An Adaptation Model* (2nd ed.), by Sister Callista Roy, pp. 42–63. Englewood Cliffs, N.J.: Prentice-Hall, Inc., 1984.

Chapter 11

Evaluation

The last step of the nursing process as described by the Roy Adaptation Model is *evaluation*. Evaluation involves judging the effectiveness of the nursing intervention in relation to the person's behavior. Was the goal that was set in the fourth step of the nursing process attained? To make this decision, the nurse assesses the behavior of the person after the interventions have been implemented. As in the initial assessment steps, the skills of observation, measurement, and interview are used. The nursing intervention would be judged effective if the person's behavior aligns with the preset goals.

Once the effectiveness of the nursing intervention has been determined, the nurse returns to the first step of the nursing process to look more closely at behaviors that continue to be ineffective.

OBJECTIVES

After studying this chapter, the reader should be able to do the following:

1. Describe the sixth step of the nursing process, *evaluation.*
2. Describe how the steps of the nursing process relate to Roy's description of the person as an adaptive system.
3. When given goal statements, describe the evidence that would indicate that nursing interventions had been effective.

4. In a given situation, evaluate the effectiveness of specific nursing interventions.

5. Identify steps to be taken when evaluation identifies ineffective results.

6. Identify steps to be taken when evaluation identifies effective results.

EVALUATION AS A REFLECTION OF GOALS

As has been discussed before, it is behavior that demonstrates the effectiveness with which the coping mechanisms are able to adapt to the stimuli affecting the person. Nursing interventions are directed towards altering stimuli in an effort to enhance the ability of the mechanisms to cope. When goals are established in step 4 of the nursing process, they are set in terms of the person's behavior and they aim to maintain and enhance adaptive behavior and to change ineffective behavior to adaptive. To evaluate the effectiveness of nursing interventions in terms of these goals, the nurse, in collaboration with the individual, must look again at the person's behavior. Have the behavioral goals been achieved? This evaluation is the sixth and final step of the nursing process. Its relationship to the previous steps and to Roy's description of the person is illustrated in Fig. 11-1.

SKILLS USED IN EVALUATION

The nurse uses the skills of observation, measurement, and interview to evaluate the effectiveness of nursing interventions as was done in the first assessment steps of the nursing process. Consider the example from Chapter 6 of the person who was hemorrhaging following surgery. Some of the ineffective behaviors identified were falling blood pressure (measured), large amount of blood on dressing (observed), and decreasing level of consciousness (observed through purposeful questioning). Goals relative to these behaviors would relate to stabilizing of blood pressure, cessation of bleeding, and regaining of consciousness, respectively. To evaluate the effectiveness of nursing interventions relative to these goals, the nurse would measure the person's blood pressure, observe the amount of blood on a fresh dressing, and use an established format for determining the level of consciousness—all skills used in making the initial assessment.

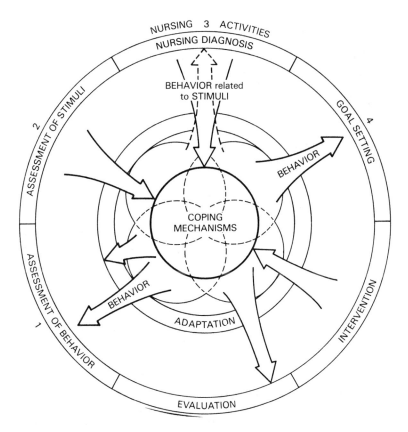

Figure 11-1   Evaluation

CONTINUITY OF THE NURSING PROCESS

For the nursing intervention to be judged effective, the person's behavior must align with the preset goals. If the goals are not achieved, the nurse must proceed to discover what went wrong. The goal may have been unrealistic or unacceptable to the person; the assessment data may have been inaccurate or incomplete; the selected approaches may not have been carried out properly. The nurse returns to the first step of the nursing process to look more closely at behaviors that continue to be ineffective.

In the example provided previously, the nurse may evaluate that the person's blood pressure has stabilized and that bleeding has stopped, but there may not be a change in the level of consciousness. Although it is still important to ensure that the stable blood pressure and cessation of bleeding are maintained, the nurse would begin to focus on the person's level of conscious and proceed through the steps of the nursing process again in order to identify an alternative approach to the ineffective behavior of decreasing level of consciousness.

Thus the nursing process is ongoing. In fact, many of the steps occur simultaneously. The nurse may be assessing behavior in one area while proceeding with a nursing intervention in another area. She may be assessing behavior and stimuli at the same time or discussing goals with the patient while she is evaluating the attainment of goals in another area.

The steps of the nursing process have been separated and specified for clarity of discussion. It is important to recognize that the nursing process is ongoing and simultaneous. It is necessary to discuss each aspect as a separate entity but one must bear in mind that each aspect is related to and affected by the other.

SUMMARY

The final step of the nursing process, evaluation, involves the assessment of the person's behavior relative to the preset goals. If the goals have been achieved, the interventions are considered to be effective; adaptive behaviors have been maintained and ineffective behaviors have been changed to adaptive. If the goals have not been achieved, the nurse must proceed to identify alternative approaches by reassessing behavior and stimuli and continuing in an ongoing and simultaneous manner with the other steps of the nursing process.

EXERCISES FOR APPLICATION

1. Assume that, as of last week, you have applied the nursing process to yourself relative to your daily diet and have set the goal that you will eat a nutritionally balanced diet containing all the recommended daily allowances for nutrients. In light of this goal, evaluate your intake of food in the past 24 hours and suggest whether your observations align with the preset goal or are ineffective in moving towards it. You may proceed through all the steps of the nursing process relative to your own situation.

ASSESSMENT OF UNDERSTANDING

Questions
1. The following paragraph is a description of evaluation as the sixth step of the nursing process as described by Roy. Underline the

word or phrase from the three in parenthesis that will complete the statement appropriately.

In evaluation, the nurse looks at the person's (coping mechanisms, behavior, stimuli) in relation to previously determined (problems, interventions, goals). The purpose of evaluation is to assess the effectiveness of (goals, nursing interventions, stimuli) in assisting the person to (adapt effectively, behave appropriately, collaborate with the nurse). If the preset goals have been achieved, the (intervention, evaluation, assessment) has been effective.

2. Label each step of the nursing process according to whether it is concerned primarily with behaviors (B), coping mechanisms (C), or stimuli (S).
   (a) _____ First level of assessment
   (b) _____ Second level of assessment
   (c) _____ Nursing diagnosis
   (d) _____ Goal setting
   (e) _____ Intervention
   (f) _____ Evaluation

3. For the following goals statements, identify what one would look for in the person's behavior that would indicate that nursing interventions had been effective.
   (a) Within one week, the patient will have regained full use of his hand as evidenced by his ability to perform a full range of motion.
   (b) By tomorrow, the patient will demonstrate increased acceptance of her role as a new mother as evidenced by her assuming responsibility for feeding and bathing of the baby.
   (c) The patient will demonstrate an understanding of the importance of the postoperative exercise regime as evidenced by the voluntary exercise every two hours following surgery.

4. The following table is a portion of information relative to a recently hospitalized four-year-old child. How would you evaluate the effectiveness of the nursing intervention? (See Table 11-1, p. 106.)

5. Relative to the situation provided in question 4, what steps should be taken relative to the ineffective behaviors identified in the evaluation step of the nursing activities?

6. The fact that the child in question 4 is beginning to relate to his roommate is an adaptive behavior even though it is not the specific behavior identified in the preset goal. What steps, if any, should be taken relative to this behavior?

Feedback
1. coping mechanisms, behavior, stimuli

TABLE 11-1   Information for Question 4

Behavior	Stimuli	Nursing Diagnosis	Goal	Interventions	Evaluation
Sitting alone in playroom Not associating with other children Crying quietly Staring at the floor Refusing to communicate with nurse	Hospitalized for the first time (contextual) Parents have just left (focal) Away from home in strange city (contextual) Does not know any of the other children (contextual)	Forlorn and upset due to separation from family	By tomorrow, the child will develop an alternative support system as evidenced by his active and happy participation with the other children in the playroom.	Take steps to increase his trust and confidence in his nurse. Introduce him to appropriate playmates. Spend time with him in playroom.	Child continues to prefer to sit alone in his room. Plays on a one-to-one basis with roommate. Asks when parents will be coming to get him.

problems, interventions, <u>goals</u>
goals, <u>nursing interventions</u>, stimuli
<u>adapt effectively</u>, behave appropriately, collaborate with the nurse
<u>intervention</u>, evaluation, assessment

2. (a) B
    (b) S
    (c) B, S
    (d) B
    (e) S
    (f) B

3. In each case, nursing interventions would be judged effective if the person was doing what was stated in the goal and in the time frame specified.

4. The goal that was set for the child has not been achieved. The behavior of continuing to sit alone in his room is ineffective if the aim is to develop an alternative support system. Playing on a one-to-one basis with his roommate is an adaptive response; the child is taking steps toward developing another support system. It is to be expected that he would ask about his parents. It is difficult to determine whether this response is adaptive or ineffective behavior with the limited information provided.

5. When ineffective behaviors are identified in the evaluation step, the nurse would proceed to step 1 to look more closely at these behaviors and the stimuli that are causing them. She may find new or different stimuli in the situation. Depending on the assessment information, it may be necessary to alter the nursing diagnosis and look again at the goal; it may have been unrealistic. Alternative nursing interventions would be assessed and then the person's behavior would be reevaluated.

6. Since the goal of nursing intervention involves the maintenance and enhancing of adaptive behaviors, it would be important that the identified adaptive responses be encouraged. They would always be considered in each step of the nursing process.

REFERENCE

Roy, Sister Callista. "The Roy Model Nursing Process," in *Introduction to Nursing: An Adaptation Model* (2nd ed.), by Sister Callista Roy, pp. 42-63. Englewood Cliffs, N.J.: Prentice-Hall, Inc., 1984.

Part IV

The Adaptive Modes

Inherent in Roy's description of the person as an adaptive system are four adaptive modes that manifest regulator and cognator activity: the physiological mode, the self-concept mode, the role function mode, and the interdependence mode. It is through these four major categories that responses are carried out and that adaptation level can be observed.

Although a definition of each of the modes was provided in Chapter 4, an overview of the model would not be complete without a more in-depth discussion of the important aspects of each of the modes. Relative to each mode are specific needs. Behaviors and stimuli that commonly influence behavior in the mode have also been identified. There are, as well, specific nursing diagnoses related to each mode.

Chapters 12 to 15 present the physiological, self-concept, role function, and interdependence modes respectively. Following a description of the components of each mode and identification of their theoretical basis, a discussion of the application of the nursing process in each of the modes is presented. It is the modes that provide the basis for a comprehensive and holistic practice of nursing and direction for the application of knowledge from related disciplines. It is not within the purpose of this text to explore this information in detail but rather to identify the applied knowledge so that the reader is aware of the theoretical basis and can pursue further information as required.

Chapter 12

The Physiological Mode

The physiological mode as described in the Roy Adaptation Model is associated with the way the person responds physically to stimuli from the environment. Behavior in this mode is the manifestation of the physiological activity of all the cells, tissues, organs, and systems comprising the human body. As with each of the adaptive modes, stimuli activate the coping mechanisms producing adaptive and ineffective behavior. In this case, the coping mechanisms are those associated with physiological functioning (primarily the regulator subsystem) and the responses produced are physiological behaviors. It is the person's physiological behavior that indicates whether the coping mechanisms are able to adapt to the stimuli affecting them.

Five needs are identified in the physiological mode relative to the basic need of physiological integrity: oxygenation, nutrition, elimination, activity and rest, and protection. Also inherent in a discussion of physiological adaptation are the complex processes involving senses, fluids and electrolytes, neurological function, and endocrine function. These can be viewed as mediating regulator activity and encompassing many physiological functions of the person.

This chapter provides the reader with an overview of the physiological mode including a description of the components of the mode and the basis for nursing assessment relative to physiological functioning. The nursing process is applied to the physiological mode with emphasis given to the assessment of behaviors and common stimuli.

OBJECTIVES

After studying this chapter, the student should be able to do the following:

1. Describe the physiological mode.
2. Identify the five needs inherent in physiological integrity.
3. Identify the four physiological components that serve as channels for the adaptive processes.

DESCRIPTION OF THE PHYSIOLOGICAL MODE

Physiology has been described as a science that deals with knowledge about the physical and chemical phenomena involved in the function and activities of a living organism. The physiological mode is the manner in which a person manifests this physiological activity. An understanding of physiological behavior necessitates a knowledge of the anatomy and physiology of the human body as well as the pathophysiology underlying disease processes. The nurse must be knowledgeable about normal body function in order to recognize behaviors that indicate problems with physiological functioning.

The underlying need of the physiological mode is *physiological integrity*. Integrity has been defined as the degree of wholeness achieved by adapting to changes in needs. When a person's physiological needs are met, physiological integrity is achieved. The Roy Adaptation Model suggests five basic needs inherent in physiological integrity: oxygenation, nutrition, elimination, activity and rest, and protection. These needs are briefly described:

1. *Oxygenation*—This need involves the body's need for oxygen and the processes of circulation and respiration, thus including the cardiovascular and pulmonary systems (Vairo 1984).
2. *Nutrition*—This need involves a series of processes associated with the ingestion and assimilation of food for maintenance of functioning, promotion of growth, and the replacement of worn or injured tissue (Servonsky 1984b).
3. *Elimination*—The need for elimination includes the physiological processes involved in the excretion of metabolic wastes primarily through the intestines and kidneys (Servonsky 1984a).
4. *Activity and rest*—A balance between physical activity and inactivity is required to provide optimal physiological functioning of all body components (Cho 1984).

5. *Protection*—The body's basic defenses include such mechanisms as immunity. The integument (skin, hair, and nails) serves an important protective function against infection, trauma, and temperature changes (Sato 1984).

In addition to the five basic needs listed above, four complex processes have been identified as important areas of consideration when assessing physiological adaptation. These processes involve the senses, fluids and electrolytes, neurological function, and endocrine function. They are viewed in the model as mediating regular activity and encompassing many physiological functions of the person.

1. *The senses*—Sight, hearing, touch, taste, and smell enable persons to interact with their environment. The sensation of pain is an important consideration in assessment of the senses (Driscoll 1984).
2. *Fluids and electrolytes*—A delicate balance of fluids and electrolytes is necessary for cellular, extracellular, and systemic function. Conversely, ineffective functioning of physiologic systems can produce electrolyte imbalance (Perley 1984).
3. *Neurological function*—Neurological channels are an integral part of a person's regulator coping mechanisms. They function to control and coordinate bodily movements and intellectual activity as well as to regulate activity of body organs and processes (Robertson 1984).
4. *Endocrine function*—Endocrine action through hormone secretion serves to integrate and coordinate body functioning. Endocrine activity plays a significant role in the stress response and is also part of the regulator coping mechanism (Howard and Valentine 1984).

These complex components of physiological adaptation together with the five basic needs described previously form the basis for physiological behavioral assessment in the Roy Adaptation Model.

THEORETICAL BASIS FOR THE PHYSIOLOGICAL MODE

The theoretical background for the physiological mode lies in the sciences of anatomy, physiology, pathophysiology, and chemistry.

1. *Anatomy*—As the study of the structure of the human body, human anatomy provides the structural basis for the physiological mode.

2. *Physiology*—Physiology provides the nurse with knowledge of the processes involved in the functioning and activities of the human body. This knowledge is the basis for judgment of adaptive and ineffective physiological behavior.

3. *Pathophysiology*—As a study of abnormal physiological changes accompanying illness, pathophysiology provides the nurse with rationale for identification of ineffective behavioral responses and the stimuli influencing them.

4. *Chemistry*—Knowledge from chemistry, dealing with the composition, properties and reactions of substances, provides the basis for an understanding of body processes such as those involved in fluid and electrolyte activity.

These sciences provide direction for some of the knowledge needed to support the study of nursing itself. As with each of the modes, consideration of the physiological mode involves application of knowledge from a variety of related disciplines. This knowledge is viewed in the light of nursing's goal of promoting adaptation.

APPLICATION OF THE NURSING PROCESS

Assessment of Behavior

Behavioral assessment of the physiological mode provides the nurse with an indication of how the person is managing to cope with environmental changes affecting the physiological coping mechanisms. Nurses are taught specific ways to conduct physical assessment of the person under their care. These methods must be thorough and yet efficient. In the Roy Adaptation Model, the basis for assessment of physiological behavior lies in the five basic needs and the four processes of physiological adaptation. These components for assessment of behavior in the physiological mode are illustrated in Table 12-1.

In the study of each of these areas, the nurse learns what behaviors reveal adaptive status in the person. The need for nutrition is used as an example.[1] The behaviors that are assessed relative to nutritional status are listed below (Servonsky 1984b):

1. Appetite and thirst
2. Height and weight

[1] The reader is directed to the definitive text (Roy 1984) for a complete discussion of physiological assessment in each of the needs and components. The scope and intent of this text does not permit such in-depth presentation.

of a nursing diagnosis stated in this manner would be, "Nutritionally inadequate diet related to insufficient resources to purchase food and lack of understanding about good nutrition." In this statement, "insufficient resources" is the focal stimulus and "lack of understanding" the contextual stimulus.

Goal Setting

The goal of nursing when applied to behavior in the physiological mode is to maintain and enhance adaptive physiological behavior and to change ineffective physiological behavior to adaptive behavior. Thus, the focus of goal setting in the physiological mode, as with any other mode, is the person's behavior.

The goal statement must consist of the three entities identified in Chapter 9: the behavior to be observed, the change expected, and the time frame for achievement of the goal. A goal related to the current example could read, "The person will plan a nutritionally adequate diet at the completion of three dietary classes."

Intervention

In order to promote adaptation, it is necessary to manage the stimuli influencing the behavior under specific considerations. It may be necessary to change the focal stimulus or to broaden the adaptation level by managing other stimuli present. In selecting approaches, the nurse considers possible alternatives and then selects the approach with the highest probability of achieving the preset goal.

Two stimuli are related to the ineffective behavior of "nutritionally inadequate diet" as identified in the example: "insufficient resources" and "lack of understanding." In this example, both stimuli must be dealt with if the person is going to achieve nutritional adequacy in his diet. For purposes of illustration, consider the selection of approaches applied to the second stimulus as depicted in Table 12-2.

The approach with the highest probability of achieving the desired results would be, "having person attend discussion-group classes on nutrition."

Evaluation

Evaluation, the final step of the nursing process, involves assessment of the person's behavior in relation to the predetermined behavioral goal. If the goal has been achieved, the intervention was effective; if not, further assessment and reconsideration of goals and intervention is required.

TABLE 12-2   Selection of Approaches as Applied to Example of Nutrition

Alternative Approaches	Consequence	Probability	Value
Alter understanding of nutrition by			
Giving person booklet on good nutrition	Enhance understanding	Moderate	Desirable
	Not enhance understanding	Moderate	Undesirable
	Confuse person	Moderate	Undesirable
Having person attend discussion-group classes on nutrition	Enhance understanding	High	Desirable
	Not enhance understanding	Low	Undesirable
Having dietary department prepare nutritionally adequate meals	Enhance understanding	Low	Desirable
	Not enhance understanding	High	Undesirable
	Person will rely on others to plan his diet	High	Undesirable

If the person in the above example is able to plan a nutritionally adequate diet after three classes on good nutrition, the preset goal has been achieved; the nursing intervention was effective.

SUMMARY

The physiological mode represents the manifestation of the person's ability to cope with changes in the environment affecting his or her physical being. Five basic needs and four adaptive processes were identified as the basis for physiological assessment. The major sciences providing the nurse with a knowledge base for nursing activities relative to the physiological mode were listed. In addition, the need for nutrition was selected to provide an example of the application of the nursing process to the physiological mode.

Figure 12-1 provides a diagrammatic representation of the nursing process as applied to the physiological mode.

Driscoll, Sheila. "The Senses," in *Introduction to Nursing: An Adaptation Model* (2nd ed.), by Sister Callista Roy, pp. 168–188. Englewood Cliffs, N.J.: Prentice-Hall, Inc., 1984.

Howard, Mary, and Sally Valentine. "Endocrine Function," in *Introduction to Nursing: An Adaptation Model* (2nd ed.), by Sister Callista Roy, pp. 238–252. Englewood Cliffs, N.J.: Prentice-Hall, Inc., 1984.

Perley, Nancy Zewen. "Fluid and Electrolytes," in *Introduction to Nursing: An Adaptation Model* (2nd ed.), by Sister Callista Roy, pp. 189–210. Englewood Cliffs, N.J.: Prentice-Hall, Inc., 1984.

Robertson, Marsha Milton. "Neurological Function," in *Introduction to Nursing: An Adaptation Model* (2nd ed.), by Sister Callista Roy, pp. 211–237. Englewood Cliffs, N.J.: Prentice-Hall, Inc., 1984.

Roy, Sister Callista. *Introduction to Nursing: An Adaptation Model* (2nd ed.). Englewood Cliffs, N.J.: Prentice-Hall Inc., 1984.

Sato, Marsha Keiko. "Skin Integrity," in *Introduction to Nursing: An Adaptation Model* (2nd ed.), by Sister Callista Roy, pp. 159–167. Englewood Cliffs, N.J.: Prentice-Hall, Inc., 1984.

Servonsky, Jane. "Elimination," in *Introduction to Nursing: An Adaptation Model* (2nd ed.), by Sister Callista Roy, pp. 125–137. Englewood Cliffs, N.J.: Prentice-Hall, Inc., 1984a.

———. "Nutrition," in *Introduction to Nursing: An Adaptation Model* (2nd ed.), by Sister Callista Roy, pp. 110–124. Englewood Cliffs, N.J.: Prentice-Hall, Inc., 1984b.

Vairo, Sharon. "Oxygenation," in *Introduction to Nursing: An Adaptation Model* (2nd ed.), by Sister Callista Roy, pp. 91–109. Englewood Cliffs, N.J.: Prentice-Hall, Inc., 1984.

Chapter 13

The Self-Concept Mode

Inherent in the description of the person as an adaptive system is the concept of holistic functioning. In viewing the person as an integrated whole, the nurse is concerned with the well-being of the total person as well as the physiological concerns discussed in the previous chapter. Ineffective behavior in any area affects the person as a whole.

The self-concept mode is one of three psychosocial modes; it focuses specifically on the psychological and spiritual aspects of the person. The basic need underlying the self-concept mode has been identified as *psychic integrity*—the need to know who one is so that one can be or exist with a sense of unity. In the process of adaptation, a person strives to achieve this psychic integrity. Adaptation problems in this area may interfere with the person's ability to heal and do what is necessary to maintain health. Thus it is important for the nurse to have knowledge about the self-concept mode in order to be able to assess behaviors and stimuli influencing a person's self-concept.

In this chapter, the self-concept mode and its components are defined and described. The theoretical basis providing direction for the assessment of behaviors and stimuli in the mode is identified and related nursing activities are presented.

OBJECTIVES

After studying this chapter, the student should be able to do the following:

1. Define *self-concept.*
2. Describe the self-concept mode together with its components.
3. Identify behaviors that manifest adaptation in the self-concept mode.
4. Identify stimuli that influence behavior in the self-concept mode.
5. When given specific behaviors and influencing stimuli, identify the nursing diagnosis that best describes them.

DESCRIPTION OF THE SELF-CONCEPT MODE

Perception of self plays a major part in everything a person does. The self-concept mode is the manifestation of behavior and level of adaptation relative to a person's beliefs and feelings about himself or herself. It is one of three modes related to psychosocial adaptation and focuses specifically on the psychological and spiritual aspects of the person. The basic need of the self concept mode is *psychic integrity.*

Self-concept has been defined as the composite of beliefs and feelings that one holds about oneself at a given time. It is formed from internal perceptions and perceptions of others' reactions. A person's self-concept directs one's behavior.

The self-concept mode is viewed in the Roy Adaptation Model as having two subareas: the physical self and the personal self. The physical self includes two components: body sensation and body image. Body sensation applies to the ability to feel and to experience oneself as a physical being. Statements such as, "I feel sick," "I feel exhausted," or "I feel great," are examples of body sensation behaviors. Body image applies to how one views oneself physically and one's appearance. "I need to lose some weight," "I feel I'm rather attractive," or "I'm not very physically fit," are all behavioral statements related to body image. Figure 13-1 is a diagrammatic representation of the self-concept with its two subareas and their components. Body sensation and body image are depicted as the two component parts of the physical self.

The personal self is viewed as having three components: self-consistency, self-ideal, and moral-ethical-spiritual self (Fig. 13-1). Self-consistency, a concept based on the work of Coombs and Snygg (1959), strives to maintain a consistent self-organization and thus avoid disequilibrium. Behavior relative to self-consistency can be observed in a person's response to a situation and his or her verbal statements: "I'm really anxious about my surgery," or "I'll be able to make a good and statement are behaviors relating to the component of the physical self, body sensation. Likewise, a person who has brought a rosary into the hospital is telling something about the moral-ethical-spiritual self. At times, it may be necessary to purposefully question a person relative to his or her self-concept. To do this effectively, the nurse must provide a comfortable and trusting environment for the person; she is asking the person to share some intimate feelings about self.

Consider the example of a girl who has been gaining weight progressively since she entered college. She wears clothes that are much too small for her and, although she was previously neatly groomed, her self-care is becoming increasingly lax. In assessing behaviors relative to her self-concept mode, the following framework is suggested and illustrated:

1. *Body sensation* (How does she feel?)—States "I don't feel attractive to others"; "I seem to have so little energy"; "I feel so fat."
2. *Body image* (How does she view herself?)—States "I'm probably a little heavy for my height"; "I don't look as good as I could just now."
3. *Self-consistency* (What is her response to the situation?)—She is slouching and appears rather dejected. Grooming has been neglected and clothes are too small. States "I'm plain and ugly."
4. *Self-ideal* (What would she like to be?)—States "I wouldn't mind losing about 70 pounds" "I'd sure like to be able to wear the size dress my sister does."
5. *Moral-ethical-spiritual self* (In what does she believe?)—States "I was probably meant to be fat"; "If I weren't fat, fate would give me some other problem."

Assessment of Stimuli

In assessing the stimuli influencing the person's behavior in the self-concept mode, the nurse again relies heavily on the theoretical basis of the self-concept as identified in the Roy Adaptation Model. To facilitate this process, six general categories of stimuli have been identified (Buck 1984). Only a brief statement about each of these factors is within the scope of this text.

1. *Perception*—This concept is based primarily on the self-perception theory of Coombs and Snygg (1959). The individual's perception of self influences the development and maintenance of a self-concept.
2. *Growth and development*—Age and degree of physical development affect one's self-concept. Known standards of growth and development provide the basis for assessment of this factor.

3. *Learning*—Based on an identified theory of learning, this concept incorporates such stimuli as societal expectations and values as well as those of significant others.

4. *Reactions of others*—This concept is based on the work of interactionists such as Cooley [Epstein (1973)], Mead (1934), and Sullivan (1953) and focuses on the influence of significant others on the person's self-concept.

5. *Maturational crises*—Based on the developmental crises identified by Erikson (1963), the age-defined developmental stage and associated maturational tasks suggest confronting challenges, achievement of which affects the person's self-concept.

6. *Coping mechanisms*—The manner in which the person characteristically functions on a day-to-day basis and in times of stress is an important stimulus influencing self-concept.

Thinking again of the example of the overweight girl, assessment information relative to stimuli may be as follows:

1. *Perception*—All statements related to how the girl sees herself apply here: "I have to work hard for my grades at school"; "My concentration span is short"; "In one word, 'fat.'"

2. *Growth and development*—She's 18 years of age, 5 feet 4 inches tall, weighs 200 pounds.

3. *Learning*—Past experiences and rewards related to learning apply: "I had top grades in secondary school and received a scholarship to this college."

4. *Reactions of others*—"I think my sister feels uncomfortable when she's in public with me"; "My parents say that 'fat' runs in the family."

5. *Maturational crises*—Identity versus role confusion is Erikson's crisis stage for an 18-year-old. The girl is studying to become a nurse: "I spend three hours each night studying."

6. *Coping mechanisms*—How does she normally deal with stressful situations? "I find I'm constantly eating when I study."

There may also be other stimuli relevant in an individual's situation and these should be included as well. Once the stimuli influencing the person's self-concept behaviors have been identified, the behaviors, in light of the theoretical bases, are judged as adaptive or ineffective in maintaining psychic integrity; stimuli are identified as focal, contextual, or residual and are labeled as to whether they are exerting a positive or negative influence on the person.

EXERCISES FOR APPLICATION

1. Formulate questions for each component of the self-concept mode (body sensation, body image, self-consistency, self-ideal, moral-ethical-spiritual self) that would be appropriate for a nurse to ask a given patient in order to elicit assessment data relative to behaviors and stimuli.

2. Interview a family member or friend to assess their self-concept and note behaviors and stimuli. Write a nursing diagnosis for each of the five components of the self-concept mode.

ASSESSMENT OF UNDERSTANDING

Questions

1. Which of the following statements apply to the *self concept* as defined in the Roy Model?
   (a) It focuses on social aspects of one's behavior.
   (b) It is a composite of beliefs and feelings about self.
   (c) It is influenced by perceptions of others' reactions.
   (d) It is one's perception of oneself.
   (e) It directs one's behavior.

2. Match the descriptions on the left with the components of the self-concept on the right. More than one description may apply.
   1. Strives to avoid disequilibrium   (a) _____ Body sensation
   2. What one would like to be   (b) _____ Body image
   3. Evaluation of who one is   (c) _____ Self-consistency
   4. The ability to feel   (d) _____ Self-ideal
   5. What one is capable of doing   (e) _____ moral-ethical-
   6. The ability to experience oneself   spiritual self
      as a human being
   7. How one views one's appearance
   8. Belief system

3. The following is a list of behaviors. Identify those that apply to the self-concept mode.
   (a) Person states "I'm so tired."
   (b) Blood pressure is 140/90 mm Hg.
   (c) Person is attractively dressed and well groomed.
   (d) Boy is slouching in chair with feet on the table.
   (e) Woman states "I really love my husband."
   (f) Person states "God has helped me through this problem."
   (g) Person calls family every evening
   (h) Person states "I'll be playing in the next game, bad knee or not."

4. List the six general categories of factors that commonly influence behavior in the self-concept mode.
   (a) _____
   (b) _____
   (c) _____
   (d) _____
   (e) _____
   (f) _____

5. Formulate nursing diagnoses for the following sets of assessment information.

Behaviors	Stimuli
Person A	
Neatly dressed.	20-year-old female, average
Appears confident.	height and weight.
"Some people might consider me	"I am confident in my abilities."
attractive."	"My family is proud of me."
"I normally feel good about myself."	Intimacy versus isolation.
"I fancy myself as an independent	
person."	
Person B	
Appears depressed.	Feels people are not interested
Reluctance to respond to questions.	in him. "Everyone ignores
"I can never do anything right."	me."
"I don't have any friends and,	"I'm not very smart."
frankly, don't really care."	"My family doesn't care what I
	do."

Feedback

1. b, c, d, e
2. (a) 4, 6
   (b) 7
   (c) 1
   (d) 2, 5
   (e) 3, 8
3. a, c, d, e, f, h
4. (a) Perception
   (b) Growth and development
   (c) Learning
   (d) Reactions of others
   (e) Maturational crises
   (f) Coping mechanisms
5. A. "Adaptive self-concept related to body image due to realistic self-perception and positive reaction from others"; or
   "High self-esteem related to positive feedback from family."
   B. "Ineffective self-concept related to self-consistency due to adverse reactions of others"; or
   "Low self-esteem related to negative feedback from significant others."

REFERENCES

Buck, Marjorie H. "Self-Concept: Theory and Development," in *Introduction to Nursing: An Adaptation Model* (2nd ed.), by Sister Callista Roy, pp. 255–282. Englewood Cliffs, N.J.: Prentice-Hall, Inc., 1984.

Coombs, Arthur, and Donald Snygg. *Individual Behavior—A Perceptual Approach to Behavior*. New York: Harper Brothers, 1959.

Driever, Marie J. "Theory of Self-Concept," in *Introduction to Nursing: An Adaptation Model*, by Sister Callista Roy, pp. 255–283. Englewood Cliffs, N.J.: Prentice-Hall, Inc., 1976.

Epstein, Seymour. "The Self-Concept Revisited or a Theory of a Theory," *American Psychologist*, 28, no. 5 (May 1973): 404–416.

Erickson, Erik H. *Childhood and Society* (2nd ed.). New York: W. W. Norton & Co., Inc., 1963.

Gardner, Bruce D. *Development in Early Childhood*. New York: Harper & Row, Publishers, 1964.

Havinghurst, Robert J. *Developmental Tasks and Education.* New York: David McKay Company, 1952.

Mead, George Herbert. *Mind, Self and Society.* Chicago: University of Chicago Press, 1934.

Roy, Sister Callista. *Introduction to Nursing: An Adaptation Model* (2nd ed.). Englewood Cliffs, N.J.: Prentice-Hall, Inc., 1984.

Sullivan, Henry Stack. *The Interpersonal Theory of Psychiatry.* New York: W. W. Norton & Co., Inc., 1953.

Chapter 14

The Role Function Mode

As emphasized previously in this book, inherent in the view of a person as an adaptive and holistic system is the understanding that problems in one area of the person's functioning will affect performance in another. In addition, people interact with other persons in groups and societies. Therefore, social adaptation is as much of a concern to the nurse as psychological and physiological adaptation.

The role function mode is one of two social modes and it focuses specifically on the roles the person occupies in society. The basic need underlying the role function mode has been identified as *social integrity* —the need to know who one is in relation to others so that one can act.

If a person is experiencing problems concerning the roles he or she occupies, the effects may be manifest in the ability to heal and maintain health. Health and illness experiences likewise affect one's role performance. For this reason, the nurse must have an in-depth knowledge about the role function mode in order to assess behaviors and influencing stimuli in the mode and to assist people in dealing with the problems they are encountering.

In this chapter, the role function mode is defined and described, the theoretical basis providing direction for assessment of behaviors and stimuli is identified, and related nursing activities are discussed.

OBJECTIVES

After studying this chapter, the student should be able to do the following:

1. Define *role*.
2. Describe the role function mode.
3. State the difference between primary, secondary, and tertiary roles.
4. State the difference between instrumental and expressive behavior.
5. Recognize partitions of instrumental and expressive behavior.
6. Identify behaviors that manifest adaptation in the role function mode.
7. Identify stimuli that influence adaptation in the role function mode.
8. Describe four common adaptation problems of the role function mode.

DESCRIPTION OF THE ROLE FUNCTION MODE

Roles have been defined as the functioning units of society (Parsons and Shils 1951). Each role exists in relationship to another. For example, the parent role requires there be a child; the employer role, an employee; and the nurse role, a patient. Associated with each role is a set of expectations about how a person behaves towards a person occupying the complementary position. Persons need to know who they are (the roles occupied) and the associated societal expectations so that they can act appropriately. This is social integrity and represents the underlying need of the role function mode.

A classification of roles as primary, secondary, and tertiary has been adopted for use in the Roy Adaptation Mode. The **primary role** determines the majority of behaviors engaged in by the person during a particular period of life. It is determined by age, sex, and developmental stage (as illustrated in Table 14-1). Examples of primary roles are 5-year-old preschool male, 16-year-old adolescent female, and 70-year-old mature adult male.

The association of age, sex, and developmental stage in labelling the primary role enables the identification of specific role behaviors in relationship to the developmental stage.

essary within the social structure to allow a person to enact role behavior, be it instrumental, (that is, goal directed) or expressive (feeling based). The four partitions constitute major stimuli for role behavior; their presence or absence permits the identification of expected behaviors for each role occupied by the person.

The partitions of behavior are (1) consumer, (2) reward, (3) access to facilities/set of circumstances, and (4) cooperation/collaboration. The following example pertaining to the sick role illustrates the application of the partitions to both instrumental and expressive behaviors.

Associated with the sick role of patient is the instrumental behavior of taking medications prescribed by another. The partitions of this behavior are as follows:

1. *Consumer*—Who or what benefits from the person's performance of role behaviors. The patient himself benefits by taking prescribed pain medication.

2. *Reward*—The rewards the individual receives for performance of role behaviors. The patient's pain is alleviated and he can increase physical mobilization.

3. *Access to facilities/set of circumstances*—The availability of materials or tools to the individual to perform role behaviors. Medication is available as is appropriate equipment for its administration.

4. *Cooperation/collaboration*—The degree to which an individual is allowed time to perform role behaviors. Medication is brought to patient. Time is allowed to elapse before its effect is felt.

There are also expressive behaviors associated with the patient role as can be noted in further application of the same four partitions:

1. *Consumer*—The need for an appropriate and receptive person to relate to for immediate feedback. Nurse is available to care for patient. Physician is actively involved in patient's care.

2. *Reward*—An established network that will provide feedback on role performance. Patient receives consistent encouragement and feedback from nurse and physician.

3. *Access to facilities/set of circumstances*—The need to feel that one has what one needs to accomplish the task. Nurse provides time to discuss patient's concerns and nursing care.

4. *Collaboration/cooperation*—The positive emotional tone and belief that the setting in which the role is performed provides the circumstances and climate needed to fulfill the role. Patient feels that he is actively involved in decisions related to his care.

THEORETICAL BASIS FOR THE ROLE FUNCTION MODE

The description of the role function mode is based on a number of specific sociological and psychological theories and principles. These provide direction for the assessment of behaviors and stimuli relative to the role function mode and, in fact, for each of the other steps of the nursing process. The following is an identification of and brief statement relative to each of the important theoretical bases of the role function mode as described in the Roy Adaptation Model.[1]

> *Goffman* (1961)—Description of role as behaviors society expects of an individual occupying a particular role.
>
> *Parsons and Shils* (1951)—Description of instrumental and expressive behaviors and the partitions associated with role interaction.
>
> *Turner* (1966)—Identification of two basic assumptions about roles; they exist in relationship to each other and are occupied by individuals.
>
> *Banton* (1965)—Identification of primary, secondary, and tertiary roles.
>
> *Erikson* (1963)—Identification of developmental tasks that provide the basis for labelling of primary role.

APPLICATION OF THE NURSING PROCESS

Assessment of Behavior

The primary, secondary, and tertiary roles the person occupies and the instrumental and expressive behaviors form the basis for behavioral assessment of social integrity relative to the role function mode. In assessing behavior in this mode, the nurse begins by identifying the person's age and related primary role. From this information, secondary roles can be projected and, by purposeful questioning, secondary and tertiary roles can be determined together with their hierarchy of importance for the person. Behavioral assessment would also include the determination of instrumental and expressive behaviors associated with each role. Direct observation of the performance of specific roles can provide further information as to adaptation in the role function mode.

Consider as an example a 19-year-old young adult female who has just entered college. In addition to the secondary role of student, one

---

[1] It is important that the reader refer to the definitive text (Roy 1984) or to the works of the identified theorists if a working knowledge of the use of these theories in the Roy Adaptation Model is sought.

can project such roles as daughter, sister, girlfriend, and participant in sports activities. Associated with the role of student are the instrumental behaviors of studying, attending classes, writing exams and papers, and participating in lab sessions. Expressive behaviors include "sounding off" with peers, complaining to parents about heavy workload, and discussing exam results with the teacher.

Following identification of the person's roles and related instrumental and expressive behaviors, tentative labels of "adaptive" and "ineffective" are applied. Adaptive behaviors are those that meet role expectations; ineffective behaviors do not meet role expectations.

Assessment of Stimuli

The four partitions of both instrumental and expressive behaviors are an important consideration when assessing stimuli influencing role function behaviors. Their presence or absence may serve as focal, contextual, or residual stimuli to the observed behaviors. Analysis of the partitions for two of the behaviors mentioned above would appear as follows:

Instrumental Behavior—Studying

1. *Consumer*—Self, significant others, teacher.
2. *Reward*—Gets good grades, passes courses, receives scholarship.
3. *Access to facilities/set of circumstances*—Library is available; evenings are reserved for study time.
4. *Cooperation/collaboration*—Teachers identify important material; boyfriend calls after 9 P.M.; classmates study at the same time.

Expressive Behavior—"Sounding Off" with Peers

1. *Consumer*—Peers.
2. *Reward*—Understanding of peers.
3. *Access to facilities/set of circumstances*—Peers have opportunity to get together after class and in residence situation.
4. *Cooperation/collaboration*—Peers are supportive of each other; all are in the same circumstances.

It is expected that a student will study; however, if one of the partitions, cooperation, is missing (boyfriend insists that the student spend all her evenings with him), it would be difficult to accomplish the prescribed behavior of studying.

In addition to the partitions, other stimuli that commonly influence behavior in the role function mode have been identified. These are listed below and illustrated with the example of the college student.

1. *Social norms*—Societal prescriptions for role behavior may vary greatly relative to culture. For example, the young woman's cultural group emphasizes the general societal expectation that students apply themselves to their study and succeed.

2. *Physical makeup and chronological age*—These influence what roles a person is suited to occupy. For example, at 19 years of age a person's learning capabilities permit study; an infant would not be occupying the role of college student.

3. *Individual's self-concept*—The person must feel capable of occupying the role. For example, the young woman feels capable of undertaking and succeeding in her selected course of study.

4. *Role models*—Their number, quality, and responses. For example, the student would look to her parents, older siblings, and other students as role models for student behaviors.

5. *Knowledge of expected behaviors*—Does the person know what behaviors are expected in performance of the role? For example, the young woman recognizes what is expected of her as a student relative to studying, obtaining passing grades, and attending class.

6. *Physical and/or emotional well-being*—This affects the individual's capacity or ability to fill the role. For example, the young woman has no physical or emotional concerns that would hinder her performance as a student.

7. *Performance in other roles*—Expectations of behavior in one role may hinder performance of behaviors in another. For example, expectations associated with the role of girlfriend could possibly infringe on prescribed student behaviors.

It is possible that stimuli other than those above are relevant in an individual's situation; these should be considered as well. Once the stimuli influencing the person's role functioning have been identified, the behaviors, in light of the theoretical bases, are judged as adaptive or ineffective in maintaining social integrity. Stimuli are identified as focal, contextual, or residual and are labelled as to whether they are exerting a positive or negative influence on the person.

Nursing Diagnosis

As was described in Chapter 8, nursing diagnosis in the role function mode involves the relating of the assessment data obtained in the first two steps of the nursing process. The label can take the form of summarizing the adaptive or ineffective behaviors related to the specific stimuli. An example of this method is, "Role mastery related to presence of all role partitions."

To assist in the labelling associated with the role function mode, four common adaptation problems have been identified:

1. *Role transition*—The process of assuming and developing a new role. It is growth in a positive direction, and is compatible with the tasks of the primary role of the individual (Nuwayhid (1984).
   (a) *Effective role transition*—The individual exhibits adaptive expressive behaviors, and a few adaptive instrumental behaviors, that partially meet with the social expectations associated with the assigned role. However, the number or quality of the behaviors is not sufficient to formulate a diagnosis of role mastery. The adaptive behaviors indicate positive movement toward the goal of role mastery (Nuwayhid 1984).
   (b) *Ineffective role transition*—The individual exhibits adaptive expressive behaviors, but ineffective instrumental behaviors for a particular role. This is usually the result of an absence of role models, and/or lack of knowledge or education for the role (Nuwayhid 1984).
2. *Role distance*—The individual exhibits both instrumental and expressive behaviors appropriate to a particular role, but these behaviors differ significantly from prescribed behaviors for the role (Schofield 1976).
3. *Role conflict*
   (a) *Intrarole conflict*—The individual fails to demonstrate instrumental and/or expressive behaviors appropriate for a role as a result of incompatible expectations concerning the individual's behavior from one or more persons in the environment (Schofield 1976).
   (b) *Interrole conflict*—The individual fails to demonstrate the instrumental and/or expressive behaviors appropriate to the individual's role as a result of occupying one or more roles that require prescribed behaviors that are incompatible with one another (Schofield 1976).
4. *Role failure*—The individual has an absence of expressive behaviors or exhibits ineffective expressive behaviors, and/or has an absence of instrumental behaviors or exhibits ineffective instrumental behaviors for a particular role (Nuwayhid 1984).

Goal Setting

Goals, set in collaboration with the person, focus on the specific role behaviors and how they will change in a given period of time. Related to the example of the college student is the following goal: "The student will increase her studying time to three hours per evening for the next week."

Intervention

As with other modes, interventions in the role function mode focus on the stimuli that are influencing the behaviors being observed. It may be necessary to change the focal stimulus or to broaden the adaptation level by managing other stimuli present by increasing, decreasing, removing, or maintaining and enhancing them. In order to increase the study time available to her, the student may have to deal with the demands her boyfriend is making. This is a change of one of the partitions for role behavior, that is, cooperation with others. Possible approaches are identified and the one with the highest probability of success is chosen for implementation.

Evaluation

As with all other modes, evaluation in the role function mode involves looking again at the preset goals to determine whether the person's behavior aligns with them.

SUMMARY

This chapter has provided an overview of the role function mode including a description and illustration of primary, secondary, and tertiary roles and the associated instrumental and expressive behavioral components. The theoretical basis for the role function mode was identified and the application of the nursing process with focus on assessment and nursing diagnosis was described. Figure 14-2 illustrates the nursing process as related to the role function mode.

EXERCISES FOR APPLICATION

1. Identify the primary, secondary, and tertiary roles in which you are currently involved.
2. Select one of your secondary roles and list the associated instrumental and expressive behaviors. Assess the partitions of one instrumental and one expressive behavior.

(f) "I have four preschool children."

7. List five stimuli that commonly influence behavior in the role function mode.

    (a) _____

    (b) _____

    (c) _____

    (d) _____

    (e) _____

8. For each of the following four statements, indicate the common role function adaptation problem they describe.

    (a) The individual exhibits adaptive expressive behaviors but ineffective instrumental behaviors when assuming a new role.

    _____ _____ _____

    (b) The individual exhibits both instrumental and expressive behaviors appropriate to a particular role, but these behaviors differ significantly from prescribed behaviors for the role.

    _____ _____

    (c) The individual fails to demonstrate the instrumental and/or expressive behaviors appropriate to the role as a result of occupation of one or more roles that require prescribed behaviors that are incompatible with one another. _____ _____

    _____

    (d) Instrumental and/or expressive behaviors are absent or ineffective for a particular role. _____ _____

Feedback

1. a, b, c

2. The role function mode is viewed as consisting of primary, secondary, and tertiary roles. Associated with each role are instrumental and expressive components, each with four associated partitions. The roles with their components and partitions form the role function mode with its basic need of social integrity—the need to know who one is in relation to others so that one can act.

3. (a) P
   (b) T
   (c) S

ASSESSMENT OF UNDERSTANDING

...estions

Which of the following statements apply to the description of *role* in the Roy Adaptation Model?

(a) It may be primary, secondary, or tertiary.

(b) It exists in relationship to another.

(c) I
(d) E
(e) E
(f) E
5. (a) 2
(b) 4
(c) 3
(d) 1
(e) 4
(f) 1
(g) 3
(h) 2
(i) 2
6. a, b, c, d, e, f
7. Any five of the following:
Presence or absence of instrumental or expressive partitions
Social norms
Physical makeup/chronological age
Individual's self-concept
Role models
Knowledge of expected behaviors
Physical and emotional well-being
Performance in other roles
8. (a) Ineffective role transition
(b) Role distance
(c) Interrole conflict
(d) Role failure

REFERENCES

Banton, Michael. *Roles: An Introduction to the Study of Social Relations*. New York: Basic Books, Inc., 1965.

Erikson, Erik H. *Childhood and Society* (2nd ed.). New York: W. W. Norton & Co., Inc., 1963.

Goffman, Erving. *Encounters*. Indianapolis: The Bobbs-Merrill Co., Inc., 1961.

Malaznik, Nancy. "Theory of Role Function," in *Introduction to Nursing: An Adaptation Model*, by Sister Callista Roy, pp. 245–264. Englewood Cliffs, N.J.: Prentice-Hall, Inc., 1976.

Nuwayhid, Kathleen Anschutz. "Role Function: Theory and Development," in *Introduction to Nursing: An Adaptation Model* (2nd ed.), by Sister Callista Roy, pp. 284–305. Englewood Cliffs, N.J.: Prentice-Hall, Inc., 1984.

Parsons, Talcott, and Edward Shils, eds. *Toward a General Theory of Action*. Cambridge, Mass.: Harvard University Press, 1951.

Randall, Brooke. "Development of Role Function," in *Introduction to Nursing: An Adaptation Model*, by Sister Callista Roy, pp. 256–264. Englewood Cliffs, N.J.: Prentice-Hall, Inc., 1976.

Roy, Sister Callista. *Introduction to Nursing: An Adaptation Model* (2nd ed.). Englewood Cliffs, N.J.: Prentice-Hall, Inc., 1984.

Schofield, Ann. "Problems of Role Function," in *Introduction to Nursing: An Adaptation Model*, by Sister Callista Roy, pp. 265–287. Englewood Cliffs, N.J.: Prentice-Hall, Inc., 1976.

Turner, Ralph H. "Role-Taking, Role Standpoint and Reference Group Behavior," in *Role Theory: Concepts and Research*, ed. Bruce Biddle and Edwin Thomas. New York: John Wiley & Sons, Inc., 1966.

Chapter 15

The Interdependence Mode

The interdependence mode is the second of two social modes identified in the Roy Adaptation Model. This mode focuses on interactions related to the giving and receiving of love, respect, and value. The basic need of this mode is termed *affectional adequacy*—the feeling of security in nurturing relationships.

Since a caring relationship is inherent in nursing activities and since persons experiencing illness have increased affectional needs, the interdependence mode is an important aspect of consideration when assessing a person's adaptive state. It is necessary for the nurse to understand the needs, behaviors, and stimuli related to this mode in order to assist patients in coping with their illness and to maintain an adaptive level of interdependence in personal relationships with others.

This chapter provides an overview of the interdependence mode consisting of a description of the mode with definitions of important terms. The theoretical basis providing direction for assessment of behaviors and stimuli is identified and related nursing activities are discussed.

OBJECTIVES

After studying this chapter, the student should be able to do the following:

1. Describe the interdependence mode.
2. Define *affectional adequacy*.
3. State the difference between *significant others* and *support system*.
4. Describe the two areas of interdependence behavior.
5. Identify behaviors that manifest adaptation in the interdependence mode.
6. Identify eight stimuli that influence adaptation in the interdependence mode.
7. Describe two common adaptation problems of the interdependence mode.

DESCRIPTION OF THE INTERDEPENDENCE MODE

Interdependence has been defined as the close relationships of people that involve the willingness and ability to love, respect, and value others; and to accept and respond to love, respect, and value given by others. It is through the social interaction of the interdependence mode that a person's need for affectional adequacy is met. Affectional adequacy, as the need underlying the interdependence mode, incorporates the need to be nurtured and to nurture and includes the needs for care and attention, affection, affirmation, belonging, approval, and understanding (Tedrow 1984).

Two specific relationships are the focus of the interdependence mode: significant others and support systems. A *significant other* is a person who is most important to the individual. Reciprocal love, respect, and value are goals inherent in the relationship. Significant others remain relatively stable for periods of time in a person's life. Under normal circumstances, significant others for a child would be the parents. A person's spouse may be classified as a significant other for many persons.

Support systems, although providing the mutual love, respect, and value inherent in relationships with significant others, differ in the intensity and meaning of the relationship. They include the other persons, individually or in groups, and possibly animals that contribute to meeting the interdependence needs of the person. Peers in the work setting may constitute a support system for an individual, as may club members, family members, friends, and pets.

relationship. The following illustrates some assessment data relative to the interdependence behavior of a 30-year-old young adult female nurse in a situation where she is caring for an 80-year-old mature adult male who has been hospitalized for a chronic illness. The focus in this situation is the patient as a significant other and the relationship is viewed from the perspective of the nurse.

Contributive Behaviors

Actively listens to gentleman's tales of yesteryear.
Holds his hand during painful procedures
Helps him prepare for meals
Ensures that he is comfortable
Checks on him frequently

Receptive Behaviors

Graciously accepts his expressions of appreciation
Is pleased to be introduced to patient's family
Accepts a candy when offered one

Following identification of the significant others and support systems and their associated behaviors, the tentative labeling of adaptive or ineffective is applied. Adaptive behaviors contribute to affectional adequacy; the relationship appears mutually satisfying. Ineffective behaviors do not contribute to affectional adequacy and there appears to be a problem in the relationship.

Assessment of Stimuli

To assist in the assessment of stimuli that influence the quality of an interdependent relationship, eight stimuli have been identified as commonly affecting interdependence behavior (Tedrow 1984). These stimuli are listed below with a brief explanation as to their significance.

1. *Need to give and receive love, respect, and value*—It is this need that causes people to form interdependent relationships. It is usually the focal stimulus in any relationship.
2. *Expectations of the relationship and awareness of needs*—Each person in an interdependent relationship must be aware of and act upon the expectations and needs of the other if the quality of the relationship is to be maintained.

3. *Nurturing ability of both persons*—The ability to nurture is thought to be directly related to experience in forming loving relationships.
4. *Level of self-esteem*—When entering relationships, people tend to associate with others having similar levels of self-esteem, a characteristic that is mutually reinforced in the relationship.
5. *Presence in the physical environment*—Physical separation makes it difficult to maintain relationships.
6. *Knowledge about friendship*—An understanding of the dynamics of friendship facilitates the building and maintaining of the same.
7. *Developmental age and tasks*—Based on Erikson (1963) and Havighurst (1953), specific age-related interdependence tasks have been identified.

Once the stimuli influencing the person's interdependent behaviors have been identified, the behaviors are judged as adaptive or ineffective in maintaining affectional adequacy and social integrity. Stimuli are identified as focal, contextual, or residual and are labeled as to whether they are exerting a positive or negative influence on the person.

In a nurse-patient relationship, problems may occur if the expectations of the relationship are not clear; the patient may expect the nurse to be doing everything for him while the nurse expects the patient to be as independent as possible. This situation would not be a mutually satisfying relationship; problems would be evident. The focal stimulus exerting a negative influence on the situation is the lack of mutual understanding of the expectations of the relationship.

Nursing Diagnosis

Formulation of a nursing diagnosis in the interdependence mode, as in any other mode, involves relating the stimuli to behaviors they are affecting either in the form of a specific statement or a generalized label encompassing typical behaviors and stimuli. A statement of nursing diagnosis indicating effective adaptation in the interdependence mode may be, "Affectional adequacy related to presence of significant other and maintenance of a mutually satisfying relationship." "Problems with a mutually satisfying relationship related to lack of mutual understanding of expectations," indicates ineffective adaptation.

To assist with the identification of ineffective behavior patterns commonly related to the interdependence mode, the following two common adaptation problems are defined.

1. *Separation anxiety*—Painful uneasiness of mind experienced by a

EXERCISES FOR APPLICATION

1. Relative to your own interdependence behavior, identify your significant others and support systems.
2. In your relationship with one significant other, identify your own contributive and receptive behaviors.
3. Formulate questions that would be appropriate for a nurse to ask a given patient in order to elicit assessment data relative to behaviors and stimuli in the interdependence mode.

ASSESSMENT OF UNDERSTANDING

Questions
1. Which of the following statements apply to the *interdependence mode*?
   (a) It relates to the psychological integrity of the individual.
   (b) It involves the giving and receiving of love, respect, and value.
   (c) It focuses on relationships with significant others and support systems.
   (d) It involves meeting needs through social interaction.
   (e) It involves nurturing relationships.
   (f) It has as its basic need the need to know who one is in relation to others.

2. Affectional adequacy, as the need underlying the interdependence mode, includes which of the following needs?
   (a) Being nurtured
   (b) Nurturing
   (c) Care
   (d) Attention
   (e) Affection
   (f) Affirmation
   (g) Belonging
   (h) Approval
   (i) Understanding

3. The following statements apply to either significant others (SO) or support systems (SS). Label each statement according to the type(s) of relationship to which it applies.
   (a) _____ Remain relatively stable for periods of time in one's life.
   (b) _____ Most important to the individual.
   (c) _____ Love, respect, and value are inherent in the relationship.
   (d) _____ Less intense and meaningful.
   (e) _____ Club members, family members, and friends are examples.

4. State the difference between receptive and contributive interdependence behaviors and provide an example of each.

5. Which of the following descriptions of behavioral data relate to the interdependence mode?
   (a) 40-year-old generative male.
   (b) Support system—extended family.
   (c) "I love my wife very much."
   (d) "Have a chocolate. My husband brought them."
   (e) "Joe has always been such a help to me."
   (f) "I really appreciate all the time you spend with me."
   (g) Occupation—teacher.

6. List the eight stimuli that were identified in this chapter as commonly influencing adaptation in the interdependence mode.
   (a) _____
   (b) _____
   (c) _____
   (d) _____
   (e) _____
   (f) _____
   (g) _____
   (h) _____

7. For each of the following statements, indicate the common interdependence adaptation problem they describe.
   (a) Painful uneasiness of mind experienced by a person who is separated from a significant other. Stages are protest, despair, and denial. _____ _____
   (b) The exceedingly unpleasant and driving experience connected with an inadequate discharge of the need for human (interpersonal) intimacy. _____

Feedback
1. b, c, d, e
2. a, b, c, d, e, f, g, h, i
3. (a) SO
   (b) SO
   (c) SO and SS
   (d) SS
   (e) SS
4. Receptive behaviors are those that indicate a person is receiving and assimilating the love, respect, and value offered by others (e.g., allowing another to hug one) while contributive behaviors are those that demonstrate giving love, respect, and value to another (e.g., hugging the other person in return).
5. b, c, d, e, f. (a and g are both roles.)

6. (a) The need to give and receive love, respect, and value
   (b) Expectations of the relationship and awareness of needs
   (c) Nurturing ability of both persons
   (d) Level of self-esteem
   (e) Level and kinds of interactional skills
   (f) Presence in the physical environment
   (g) Knowledge about friendship
   (h) Developmental age and tasks
7. (a) Separation anxiety
   (b) Loneliness

REFERENCES

Brown, Sue Ann. "Loneliness," in *Introduction to Nursing: An Adaptation Model* (2nd ed.), by Sister Callista Roy, pp. 442–457. Englewood Cliffs, N.J.: Prentice-Hall, Inc., 1984.

Erikson, Erik M. *Childhood and Society*. New York: W. W. Norton & Co. Inc., 1963.

Fromm, Eric. *The Art of Loving*. New York: Harper & Row, Publishers, 1956.

Havighurst, R. T. *Human Development and Education*. New York: Longmans, Green & Co., 1953.

Randell, Brooke, Mary Tedrow, and Joyce VanLandingham. *Adaptation Nursing: The Roy Conceptual Model Made Practical*. St. Louis: The C. V. Mosby Co., 1982.

Roy, Sister Callista. *Introduction to Nursing: An Adaptation Model* (2nd ed.). Englewood Cliffs, N.J.: Prentice-Hall, Inc., 1984.

Selman, R. C. *The Growth of Interpersonal Understanding: Development and Clinical Analysis*. New York: Academic Press, Inc., 1980.

Servonsky, Jane, and Mary Poush Tedrow. "Separation Anxiety," in *Introduction to Nursing: An Adaptation Model* (2nd ed.), by Sister Callista Roy, pp. 428–441. Englewood Cliffs, N.J.: Prentice-Hall, Inc., 1984.

Tedrow, Mary Poush. "Interdependence: Theory and Development," in *Introduction to Nursing: An Adaptation Model* (2nd ed.), by Sister Callista Roy, pp. 306–322. Englewood Cliffs, N.J.: Prentice-Hall, Inc., 1984.

Part V

The Roy Adaptation Model in Nursing Practice

The Roy Adaptation Model has been described throughout this text as a systematic framework for nursing activities. That is, it guides the activities of the nursing process which include assessment, nursing diagnosis, goal setting, intervention, and evaluation.

Nursing models have been used as the basis for the curriculum of formal nursing education. Their use in the practice setting will help to align what is done in nursing practice with what is taught in nursing education and will help to enhance the quality of care provided by the nurse.

The following section describes applications of the Roy Adaptation Model in the practice setting. It demonstrates how nursing models and the Roy Model in particular are beginning to be used in practice. Written from the perspective of a nursing inservice education director and a clinical nurse specialist in an acute-care pediatric hospital, the intent of this section is to encourage nurses to consider the patient care ramifications of the implementation of a nursing model in their own practice setting.

Chapter 16

The Roy Adaptation Model in Nursing Practice

Maureen T. Jakocko, Master of Nursing

Linda A. Sowden, Master of Nursing

Historically, nursing has been viewed as an art and a science. In caring for the sick and helping others stay well, nurses have skillfully based their activities on tradition, previous experience, and the application of phenomena from related sciences. The *science of nursing* itself is in the developing stages. Nursing is identified as a science in that phenomena are observed and classified, relationships are established, and interactions are stated and tested (Roy 1984).

Over the past few decades, nursing models have been developed to provide a basis for the development of the science of nursing. Nursing models provide a representation of how particular nurses describe nursing science's view of persons, environment, nursing, and health in order to clarify what nursing is and what services nurses can provide. The result is a systematic development of nursing knowledge as the scientific basis for nursing practice.

Nursing as a scientific discipline is practice oriented; the ultimate focus of discussion and thought is the practice setting—the point where nurse and patient interact to achieve their health-related goals. A scientific approach to nursing based on a conceptual model enables the nurse to identify consistently effective approaches to patient concerns. What is learned in one situation can be tested in another, ultimately generating new knowledge to positively affect health in understandable and consistent ways.

Since nursing as a science is currently in the developing stages, nurses in the practice setting are functioning with a diversity of frameworks. This situation has caused a variety of problems: vocabularies vary, there is a lack of definition and direction for nursing activities, and inconsistencies in patient care develop. The commitment by nurses to the use of one conceptual model for nursing in a practice setting helps to alleviate these problems and ultimately enhances the quality and consistency of patient care.

The following is a description of how one nursing model, the Roy Adaptation Model, has been applied in the practice setting both at the patient's bedside and from the administrative point of view.

THE ROY ADAPTATION MODEL IN PRACTICE

The use of the Roy Adaptation Model in nursing practice has been described in inpatient, outpatient, and community settings. There has been further documentation as to its utility in nursing service administration at both the National Hospital for Orthopedics and Rehabilitation in Arlington, Virginia, and at the Childrens Hospital of Orange County in Orange, California. A compilation of specific examples of the application of the model was described by Fawcett (1984).

The Roy Adaptation Model has many applications in planning for and delivering care using the nursing process. The model provides the nurse with a systematic framework for assessment and for planning and implementing interventions. As the model has become increasingly used in patient care, implications for nursing administration are becoming evident and theoretical explorations are beginning to be applied.

THE ROY ADAPTATION MODEL IN PATIENT CARE

As presented throughout this text, the Roy Adaptation Model has many applications in planning for and delivering patient care. The model provides a framework for assessment, for planning interventions after specific concerns have been identified, and for evaluating effectiveness of preset goals.

Upon the patient's admission to an acute-care facility or outpatient clinic, the nurse begins care for the patient by obtaining a detailed patient history as part of the initial assessment. It is important that such a history be obtained by interview as it provides the opportunity to establish rapport and creates an open environment in which the patient can share information regarding physical condition, feelings, and concerns (Koeckeritz 1981). The Roy Adaptation Model, as a systematic approach to assessing adaptation, lends structure to the patient history interview.

Age-related patient admission history/assessment forms were developed at Childrens Hospital of Orange County by members of the nursing staff. (See Appendix 1.) All four modes are assessed. After demographic data are obtained, the assessment of current and relevant past behaviors begins. This includes those behaviors that are reported, observed, and measured.

Each category of the physiological mode is assessed:

1. *Oxygenation*—Oxygenation is assessed by heart and respiratory rates with corresponding quality and rhythm, observation of color, report of dyspnea, hemoptysis, and cough.
2. *Nutrition*—A nutritional history is obtained which includes type of diet, mealtimes, food preferences, and special considerations such as allergies.
3. *Elimination*—Elimination is assessed by obtaining information regarding bowel and bladder habits.
4. *Activity and rest*—Activity and rest are assessed by sleep patterns, bedtime routines, sleep position, motor development, and favorite toys.
5. *Protection*—Skin integrity is assessed by observing overall condition including rashes and bruises. At this time, a history of skin sensitivities is obtained, as well.
6. *Senses*—The senses are assessed by determining visual and auditory acuity and presence and kind of pain or loss of feeling.
7. *Fluids and electrolytes*—When assessing fluids and electrolytes, the hydration status is observed along with the time of last oral fluids, void, and stool.
8. *Neurological function*—Neurological function is assessed by the patient's level of consciousness, muscle tone, and gross and fine motor skills. History of trauma or disorders is noted.
9. *Endocrine function*—Endocrine function is assessed by observing structural and functional development such as stature, sexual development, and history of endocrine imbalance (hyper- or hypoglycemia, for example).

Included in the assessment of the self-concept mode are temperament, fears, response when upset, and past hospitalization experiences. The role function mode is assessed by obtaining information regarding those who live in the home, siblings, and special activities. The interdependence mode is assessed by learning if the child, for example, has been away from parents before, who the primary caretaker is, and any recent changes at home.

Following the initial admission assessment, the nurse continues to assess the patient as nursing care is planned and provided. An ongoing physiological assessment and record of nursing care in the format of a 24-hour flow sheet was developed at Childrens Hospital of Orange County. When the oxygenation category is assessed, vital signs are recorded along with an assessment of color, respiratory quality, and circulation. Treatments related to oxygenation (suctioning, for example) are charted when given. Comments about intravenous sites and restrained extremities are made in the skin category along with documentation of skin care given.

When assessing activity and rest, patient activity and positioning are recorded. Included in the neurological category is an assessment of level of consciousness, pupils, handgrip, and leg movement. Finally, the nutrition, elimination, and fluid and electrolyte categories are divided into intake and output. Intake includes an assessment of the amount and type of diet eaten, oral fluids, and a record of the amount and type of parenteral fluid infused. Output includes the amount of urine and stool output, emesis, and catheter drainage.

When planning for discharge, the Roy Adaptation Model serves as a framework for the systematic identification of discharge needs in order to provide continuity of care between the hospital and home. The goals of discharge planning are to ensure that (1) the patient and his or her family have adequate information for care at home, (2) the patient will receive the health care needed without interruption, and (3) information is shared with other agencies so that care is not interrupted (Peabody 1972).

The process of discharge planning involves the application of the nursing process relative to each of the four modes. Physiologically, each category is reviewed to identify specific needs to be addressed prior to discharge—patient education, special equipment, follow-up care, and medication. The psychosocial modes are assessed by identifying the need for assistance in the home and the relevance of and need for support groups (Hoffmans 1979). After identifying discharge needs, the nursing process continues with goal setting and interventions. Evaluation criteria for discharge are established according to the model. The following situation serves as an example.

Wendy Ryan, a three-month-old, is to be discharged with a tracheostomy. Her discharge needs in the area of oxygenation include the need for obtaining special equipment such as a suction machine and catheters, extra tracheostomy supplies, and humidified air to be delivered via tracheostomy collar. Her mother needs specific education in the operation, care, and maintainance of the equipment along with instruction in suctioning technique, changing the tracheostomy and ties, and signs, symptoms, and management of complications including cardio-pulmonary resuscitation.

Intradisciplinary patient care conferences provide the health-care team with the opportunity to collaborate in identifying problems and planning potential treatment. Since each discipline operates from a different framework, the conference requires organization in order to be productive. The Roy Adaptation Model, with its holistic, biopsycho-social view of the person, provides an excellent framework for the conference. The four modes provide a structure in which participants from each discipline may discuss their particular areas of involvement.

In situations where patient education is identified as a need, content must be systematically organized in order to be understood by the patient. The Roy Adaptation Model can be used as a framework for the lesson plan. Judd (1983) used the model to organize content when teaching patients about congestive heart failure.

The above discussion illustrates how the Roy Adaptation Model can be applied in the patient care situation. It is to be anticipated that innovative ways to apply the model will be identified as more practice settings begin to use the model as their basis for nursing practice. Implications for the area of nursing administration are being identified in settings where the model has been implemented in practice, as illustrated in the following discussion.

THE ROY ADAPTATION MODEL IN NURSING ADMINISTRATION

Although much of the discussion of the application of the Roy Adaptation Model is in the theoretical stage, some progressive developments are beginning in the application of ideas in nursing administration departments. There is potential for a nursing model to become the common denominator that unifies the department of nursing; its applicability is evident in such aspects as standards of care, inservice education, course curriculum, job descriptions, employee evaluation tools, employee counselling, patient classification systems, and computer technology.

Nursing, as a profession, is accountable for care rendered to patients. Standards of care help to accomplish this task. In Bolinger et al. (1979) standards of care based on the Roy Adaptation Model were developed for preschool-age children admitted to the hospital for repair of patent ductus arteriosus. In a hospital with standards of care written by various staff members, a nursing model gives direction and serves as a framework to be followed.

The Roy Adaptation Model has been used in developing course curricula for nursing inservice education. As the result of an assessment of the educational needs of the nursing staff on the oncology unit at Childrens Hospital of Orange County, a comprehensive course based on the Roy Adaptation Model was developed. The course content was divided into physiological, self-concept, role function, and interdependence modes. Topics such as physiological assessment, physical nursing interventions, growth and development, stressors of hospitalization, the child's concept of death, and the impact and effect of diagnosis on the family were included.

Job descriptions and employee performance tools may be developed using the Roy Adaptation Model. In a job description, the model helps to outline in a complete, orderly fashion the Department of Nursing's expectations of the nurse's role. Orientation and annual appraisals include an evaluation of the nursing care provided using the four adaptive modes. Hence, comprehensive care of the patient is assured.

Employee counselling is another area where the model has been used in nursing administration. After attending a class on the Roy Adaptation Model, a charge nurse used her knowledge and creativity to develop a method of counselling an employee (Doerr 1983). Ineffective behaviors were identified along with focal, contextual, and residual stimuli. The problem was identified, measurable goals stated, and interventions defined. The employee was evaluated within the time frame stated in the goal for behavior change.

Classification systems document care requirements according to the acuity of patients' conditions and thereby justify staffing patterns. Traditionally, acuity systems have been based on the physiological aspects of care. An acuity system based on the Roy Adaptation Model is an effective tool. Both physiological and psychosocial needs are identified using the four modes. Patients are categorized according to need based on the assessment of the entire person. Such problems as anxiety, role transition, and loneliness are now being taken into account in the ranking of the patient.

In this age of computers, many hospitals are preparing for their use in various tasks. The Roy Adaptation Model can be used for organizing information to be programmed into the computer. It could provide a vocabulary, continuity, and structure for the task.

The above discussion represents but the beginning steps in the application of the Roy Adaptation Model in nursing administration. As was true in the area of patient care, innovative applications of the model will be forthcoming as its use in nursing service administration increases.

CONCLUSION

The potential of the Roy Adaptation Model, or any other nursing model, will be realized only as increased numbers of nurses collectively make the decision to base their practice on such a conceptual framework. The communication of ideas, successes and failures, problems and solutions, both by word of mouth and in print, cannot be stressed enough. All contribute to the development of the science of nursing. It is hoped that this discussion will encourage practicing nurses to evaluate the elements of the model as presented in this text relative to their own beliefs and the situation in their practice setting with a view to applying it as the basis for nursing and then to share their experiences with other concerned nurses.

REFERENCES

Bolinger, T., J. Golonka, M. Jakocko, C. Purzycki, and L. Sowden. "Standards of Care Based on the Roy Adaptation Model," Course Requirements, U.C.L.A. Graduate School of Nursing, November 19, 1979.

Doerr, S. Personal communication, July 13, 1983.

Fawcett, J. *Analysis and Evaluation of Conceptual Models of Nursing.* Philadelphia: F. A. Davis, 1984.

Hoffmans, M. A. "Discharge Planning Manual," Childrens Hospital of Orange County, Orange, Calif., September 1979.

Judd, C. Personal communication, October 21, 1983.

Koeckeritz, J. "How to Coax out a Frank Patient History," *R.N.*, October 1981, pp. 57-61.

Peabody, S. R. "Assessment and Planning for Continuity of Care from Hospital to Home," *Nursing Clinics of North America*, 4 (June 1969): 303.

Roy, Sister Callista. *Introduction to Nursing: An Adaptation Model* (2nd ed.). Englewood Cliffs, N.J.: Prentice-Hall, Inc., 1984.

Admission History/Assessment
Childrens Hospital of
Orange County

Childrens Hospital of Orange County

Orange, California

Admission History/Assessment
Age: Infant/Toddler (0-2½ years)

Primary Nurse _____ Admitting Nurse _____

Admission Notes: Date _____ Time _____ Room _____ Language _____

T ___ AP ___ R ___ B/P ___ HC ___ HT ___ (cm) WT ___ (Kg) Age ___

Mode of Transportation/Accompanied by: _____

Reason for admission: _____

History of illness and pertinent information: _____

_____

_____

Physiological Mode
1. Oxygenation

a. Pulse quality and rhythm: ☐ Regular ☐ Irregular

Comments: _____

b. Respiratory quality: ☐ Clear ☐ Equal ☐ Unlabored

Comments: _____

c. Special considerations (O_2, cyanosis, diaphoresis, trach. monitors, etc.): _____

2. Fluid and Electrolytes

a. Abnormal fluid losses (diarrhea, vomiting, etc.): _____

b. Hydration: Last void _____ Last P.O. _____ Skin turgor: ☐ Good ☐ Fair ☐ Poor

Tearing: ☐ yes ☐ no   Mucous membranes: ☐ Moist ☐ Dry ☐ Tacky

Comments (edema, weight changes, etc.): _____

3. Skin Integrity

a. Previous problems with temp. maintenance: _____

b. Overall condition: ☐ Clear   Comments (rash, bruises, scars, etc.): _____

c. Special considerations (wounds, breakdown, etc.): _____

4. Neurological

a. Fontanels: ☐ Flat ☐ Soft ☐ Full ☐ Bulging ☐ Depressed ☐ Closed

b. Level of consciousness: ☐ Alert ☐ Lethargic   Comments: _____

c. History of trauma or disorders (shunts, hyper/hypotonia, etc.): _____

5. The Senses

a. Vision: ☐ Normal   Hearing: ☐ Normal   Speech: ☐ Normal

b. Special considerations: _____

6. Nutrition

a. ☐ Milk ☐ Breastfed ☐ Formula   Type _____ Amount _____ Temp. _____ Schedule _____

Type of bottle/nipple: _____

b. Diet: ☐ Purees ☐ Junior ☐ Finger ☐ Table   Started: ☐ Whole eggs ☐ Orange juice

c. Schedule: _____ Favorite foods/drinks: _____

d. Special considerations (N/G, GER, etc.): _____

e. Takes medication best: _____

7. Elimination

a. Potty trained: ☐ yes ☐ no   Words used _____ Last BM _____

b. Special considerations (crede, catheter, laxative, etc.): _____

8. **Activity and Rest**
   a. Usual hours of nighttime sleep: _____ Naptime Hours: _____
   b. Bedtime routine: _____
   c. Where does child sleep? _____ Sleep position: _____
   d. What is done for sleeplessness? _____
   e. Motor development: ☐ Rollover ☐ Sits ☐ Crawls ☐ Stands ☐ Walks
      ☐ Other _____
   f. Where does chld usually spend the day? _____
   g. Favorite toys (blanket, etc.): _____
   h. Car seat: ☐ yes ☐ no

9. **Endocrine**
   a. Structural (stature, sexual development, etc.): _____
   b. Functional (Hyper/hypo thyroid, diabetes, etc.): _____

Psychosocial Modes

1. **Self-Concept**
   a. Nicknames: _____
   b. Describe child's usual temperament: _____
   c. Child's response when held: ☐ Relax ☐ Stiffens ☐ Cuddles
   d. Fears (dark, noises, strangers, etc.): _____
   e. Child's response when upset (breathholding, bites, kicks, etc.): _____
   f. Previous hospital experiences: _____
   g. Hospital preparation: ☐ Pre-op party   Other: _____

2. **Role Function**
   a. Siblings (names and ages): _____
   b. Who lives in the home with the patient? _____ Pets: _____
   c. Who will visit? _____ Participation: _____
   d. Parenting classes: ☐ yes ☐ no

3. Interdependence

a. Primary caretaker: _____

b. Has child been away from parents? ☐ yes ☐ no   With whom: _____

   Frequency: _____   Reaction: _____

c. Recent changes at home (death, separation, moving, etc.): _____

   Reaction: _____

d. Methods of comforting (voice, hold, rock, etc.): _____

e. Pacifier: ☐ yes ☐ no   Thumb/finger sucking: ☐ Right ☐ Left ☐ Bilateral ☐ None

f. Will someone spend the night? ☐ yes ☐ no   Who? _____

g. Parental concerns with hospitalization: _____

h. Visitation or transportation problems: _____

i. Special programs/agencies involved with child/family (PHN, CCS, Rehab., etc.): _____

Family Orientation

☐ Room
☐ Bedrails/Bed
☐ Call light/TV
☐ Telephone

☐ Visitors' policy
☐ Overnight stays
☐ Isolation
☐ Daily Routines

☐ Tub/shower
☐ Meals
☐ Kitchen
☐ Parents' lounge

☐ Restrooms
☐ Cafeterias
☐ Playroom
☐ Wagons/strollers

☐ Linen
☐ Diapers
☐ I&O/Bottles
☐ Letter
☐ Breast pump

Index

A

Access to facilities, role partition, 139
Acquired coping mechanisms, 21, 38
Activity (*See* Activity and rest)
Activity and rest, 80, 112, 167, 168
Adaptation:
  defined by Helson, 8
  goal of nursing, 51
  health, 50
  indicators, 62
Adaptation difficulty, indication, 60, (*See* Adaptation problem)
Adaptation level, 21, 30-32, 91, 92
  definition, 30
Adaptation problem:
  common, 78-80
  definition, 77
  (table), 80

Adaptive, definition, 22
Adaptive behavior, 6, 32
  judgement, 60-61
Adaptive modes, 7, 41-44, 109
  and coping mechanisms, 37, 41
  interdependence, 43, 151-158
  physiological, 41-42, 111-118
  role function, 42-43, 135-144
  self-concept, 42, 123-130
Adaptive responses (*See* Adaptive behavior)
Adaptive system:
  goals, 21
  person as, 6, 18-22
Adequacy, affectional, (*See* Affectional adequacy)
Admission history/assessment, 167
Affectional adequacy, 43, 152
Aggressive sexual behavior, 80
Anatomy, 113
Anxiety, 80
Application of Roy Adaptation Model:
  nursing administration, 169